P9-AGA-170

DATE DUE

NO 18 '94			
RENEW			
DE 9 '94			
AP 17 '95			
NO 19 '96			
NOV 26 1996			
OC 20 '97			
DE 2 '97			
FE 19 '98			
MR 10 98			
MR 22 '99			
DE 7 '99			
DE 29 '99			
AP 15 02			
JR 17 05			
FE 23 '08			

DEMCO 38-296

IMMUNE
POWER

The

Comprehensive

Healing

Program

for

H I V

JON D. KAISER, M.D.

IMMUNE POWER

Combining Holistic and

Standard Medical

Therapies into the Optimal

Treatment Program for

HIV

St. Martin's Press New York

Riverside Community College
Library
4800 Magnolia Avenue
AUG '99 Riverside, California 92506

IMMUNE POWER. Copyright © 1993 by Jon D. Kaiser,
M.D. All rights reserved. Printed in the United States
of America. No part of this book may be used or re-
produced in any manner whatsoever without written
permission except in the case of brief quotations em-
bodied in critical articles or reviews. For information,
address St. Martin's Press, 175 Fifth Avenue, New
York, N.Y. 10010.

Design by Judith A. Stagnitto

Library of Congress Cataloging-in-Publication Data

Kaiser, Jon D.
    Immune power : a comprehensive healing program
for HIV / Jon D. Kaiser.
        p.   cm.
    ISBN 0-312-09312-8
    1. AIDS (Disease)—Treatment. 2. AIDS (Dis-
ease)—Alternative treatment. 3. Holistic medicine.
I. Title.
RC607.A26K35   1993
616.97'9206—dc20   93680
                                              CIP

10 9 8 7 6 5 4 3 2

To my patients,

whose commitment and dedication to healing

provides me with a continual source of inspiration.

CONTENTS

Author's Note   / *ix*

Preface   / *xi*

1. Viral Dormancy   / *1*

2. Private Practice Data   / *11*

3. Natural Therapies   / *17*
   - Diet
   - Vitamins and Nutritional Supplements
   - Herbs
   - Exercise
   - Stress Reduction

4. Emotional Healing   / *79*
   - The Importance of Growth
   - Specific Techniques
   - Letters to the Virus

5. Standard Medical Therapies   / *121*
   - Lab Tests
   - Antiviral Drugs
   - Prophylaxis
   - Treatment of Cofactors
   - Treatment of Specific Symptoms and Conditions
   - Experimental Therapies

6. Case Histories: Examples of Viral Dormancy / 192

*Appendix: Comprehensive Healing Program
for HIV-Research Study* / 206

Notes: For Study Results / 218

References / 220

Stress Reduction and Positive Affirmation Tapes / 228

Index / 229

AUTHOR'S NOTE

The Immune Power protocol is based on the experiences and observations of the author. It is meant to provide information to educate patients and their physicians on how to integrate both alternative and standard medical therapies in the treatment of HIV and other immune system disorders. The natural therapy and emotional healing aspects of this program are designed to be an adjunct to, not a substitute for, conventional medical therapy.

No treatment program, whether it be alternative, conventional, or a combination of the two, is effective for everyone. Some people may become worse despite any therapies or lifestyle changes. The goal of this book is to provide a program that will help many people improve the status of their health and significantly delay the progression of their condition. It is extremely important that no changes in your medical program be made without first conferring with your doctor.

Finally, I feel it is important to state that although many products and companies are mentioned throughout this book as possessing high quality and good value, the author has not received any monetary compensation or other gratuitites from any of them.

PREFACE

Five years ago, when I opened my private practice, I believed that *a comprehensive approach to the treatment of AIDS* would be more effective than the medical regimen currently prescribed as the community standard.

I define a comprehensive approach as one which adds a program of *natural therapies* and *emotional healing techniques* to the standard medical treatment of a given illness or condition. A natural-therapies program includes a combination of diet, vitamins, herbs, exercise, and stress reduction. Emotional healing encompasses a proactive program of psychological healing techniques that ideally includes an emotional-support group.

In theory, adding a program of natural therapies to the best that standard medical therapy has to offer will always improve the result beyond what might be achieved utilizing either approach alone. Until modern medicine places enough emphasis on the use of nutrition, vitamins, stress reduction, and other natural healing techniques as part of its recommended program of therapies, it will always fall short of achieving the best possible result. This book is designed to help both patients and practitioners integrate these two approaches.

It is important to realize that AIDS is not a gay disease. AIDS is not a disease that only affects men. AIDS is not a disease of adults, whites, or blacks. AIDS is a disease that will, increasingly over time, span all geographic and cultural boundaries. Its outstretched hand will affect forty million people by the end of this decade.

Because of these facts, it is important for the world's research community to focus on finding treatments that will work for all people regardless of their age, race, or sexual orientation.

I myself admit that I am guilty of focusing my research efforts, to date, exclusively on one social group, gay men. I am guilty with an explanation, however. Gay men were the only individuals who volunteered to participate in my study when it began in 1987. In the future, I plan to actively recruit from many different socio-economic groups for individuals to participate in my research projects.

It is strongly recommended that, unless you are extremely familiar with interpreting HIV-related lab tests, you should first read the Lab Tests section of the Standard Medical Therapies chapter. This will simplify your understanding of what T-cells are and how they influence the decisions an individual needs to make throughout the course of living with HIV.

It has taken five years to compile the information presented in this book. While following this path, I have learned many interesting facts. First, I have learned that an individual's emotions play an integral part in the progression of, and in healing from, any illness. Secondly, I have learned that when drugs are added to an aggressive natural therapies program, they can be utilized in lower dosages to achieve the same results that they normally would have achieved when used at higher dosages alone. Utilizing medications in this fashion allows a patient to experience the drug's positive benefits while reducing undesirable side effects.

I would sincerely like to thank the following people and organizations for their help in bringing this project to fruition: Claire Hangen; Carolyne Waite; Timothy Tafoya; Dr. Laurence Badgley; Dr. Dean Ornish; Dr. Linus Pauling; Dr. Keith Barton; Randall Leonard; Wil Garcia; George Melton; Charlie Swanson; Ilana Goldner; Steven Sparler; Sadie McFarlane; Jane and Steve Restaino; Michael Denenny; George Greenfield; Bruce, Beth and Max Hollander; Joan and Alex Kaiser, my parents; and my entire family.

Also, very special thanks to Twin Laboratories, Inc.; Pacific Biologic, Inc., KAL, Inc.; Dr. Elizabeth Donegan; Vilma Remedios; Paula Pell; the Transfusion Safety Study staff; and the Comprehensive Healing Program Research Study Group for their invaluable assistance.

I would also like to thank my colleagues at the San Francisco Community Consortium, including its director, Donald Abrams,

M.D., and its staff. This group of men and women has worked tirelessly on the front lines of the war against AIDS during the past several years. Their goal has been to provide quality AIDS education and treatment to all those who need it, and they have succeeded admirably in this endeavor. They have been particularly successful in setting up community-based trials to provide the data necessary for speeding the progress of beneficial therapies from the research arena into general use. I am proud to be associated with this fine organization.

And finally, a tip of the hat to a true Jedi healer, my friend and confidant, Ms. Peggy Flynn.

IMMUNE
POWER

One

VIRAL DORMANCY

*"In wisdom we look at the whole, in
ignorance we look at the parts."*

Plato

During the past decade, AIDS has become an immense global
problem. The World Health Organization estimates that between
eight and ten million people worldwide are currently infected with
the Human Immunodeficiency Virus (HIV). It is estimated that
by the year 2000, forty million people worldwide will be infected.
Many, if not all, of these individuals will eventually be diagnosed
with AIDS.

In the United States alone, over two thirds of the 210,000
patients who have been diagnosed with AIDS have died.* In spite
of several important medical advances, including the use of AZT
and aerosol pentamadine, thousands of people continue to experience a progressive decline in the strength of their immune systems. This experience clearly illuminates the fact that the medical

---

*The definition of AIDS used in this book is based on the 1987 CDC criteria
which require a previous incidence of an opportunistic infection or the presence of Kaposi's sarcoma.

establishment's current approach to the treatment of this condition is inadequate. Unless a more effective treatment approach is found, the majority of these infected individuals will eventually become sick and die—sending a ripple of pain, suffering, and economic hardship throughout our entire society.

A NEW MODEL

If we accept the current medical paradigm, which states that infections are "caused" by microscopic bacteria, viruses, and fungi that invade the body, regardless of a person's diet and lifestyle, then HIV is treated as an "invader" which must be destroyed at all costs. This entices the physician, and the patient, to believe that drugs are the only answer for its treatment. However, it is clearly seen that most patients who utilize drugs *as the sole means for their HIV treatment* continue to experience a gradual yet inevitable decline in the strength of their immune systems. It is therefore necessary for us to develop a more effective treatment model to help keep those infected alive and productive after they initially test positive for exposure to HIV.

HIV is a retrovirus. Accordingly, it enters your cell as a piece of RNA (ribonucleic acid), replicates into a new piece of DNA (deoxyribonucleic acid), and then incorporates itself into your own cell's DNA. Because of this, there is no way, theoretically or practically, to extricate it from the genetic code of your cells once it has incorporated itself. If the standard medical approach is followed, namely to poison the infective agent with drugs, a high risk is run of damaging your own cells' DNA in the process. This is why antivirals such as AZT, in high doses, can be so toxic. They work to inhibit the replication of your own cells' DNA in the same way that they attempt to inhibit the replication of the HIV virus's DNA.

The Comprehensive Healing Program for HIV, in addition to utilizing standard medical therapies such as antivirals, especially focuses on maintaining a strong host resistance to disease. To accomplish this, *a natural therapies program,* including healthful recommendations on diet, vitamins, herbs, exercise, and stress reduction, is *added* to the currently recommended standard medical approach. When natural therapies are used in combination with standard medical therapies, a much more effective treatment plan emerges. It has been my experience that this combination approach is absolutely necessary if the treatment of HIV is to be successful.

ACHIEVING VIRAL DORMANCY

Dr. William A. Haseltine, chief of the Human Retrovirology Department at Harvard Medical School, has described in detail the factors that regulate the activity of HIV once it has become incorporated into the human cell. In a paper presented at the December 1990 AIDS Care Symposium in San Francisco, Dr. Haseltine stated, "In T-cells, HIV can lie dormant indefinitely, inextricable from the cell but hidden from the victim's immune system." He went on to say, "The intricate mechanisms for controlling HIV's growth do not operate in isolation; they are intimately intertwined with the physiology of the host cell . . . the host cell, through its array of transcription factors, creates a molecular environment that influences the working of HIV's own regulatory mechanisms."

Once HIV has incorporated itself into your cells, the only way to eliminate its negative effects is by encouraging it to become dormant. HIV dormancy is an achievable phenomenon. It is the condition in which the genes that instruct HIV to replicate itself are quiescent. Your cells then, by definition, are unaffected by the virus's presence.

The genetic switch for viral growth is found on the HIV genome in the form of three regulatory genes. These are the "tat" (transactivator), "rev" (regulator of virion-protein expression) and "nef" (negative regulatory factor) genes. The importance of these genes lies in their ability to determine the activity level of HIV inside the cell. Dr. Haseltine states that "individually or through their interplay, [these genes] can specify explosive viral replication, moderate growth, or quiescence."

HIV can enhance or depress its own level of activity. It can therefore be totally active or completely dormant. The ability of a virus to so closely regulate its own expression, based on the conditions of its intracellular environment, indicates that it is a highly evolved organism. It is able to assess its environment and react accordingly.

Dr. Haseltine has postulated a reason for the evolution of this trait. "Because controlled growth enables a virus to reproduce itself for years without killing off its host . . . such genetic regulation may be an adaptive feature for any retrovirus that infects a long-lived species such as human beings."

Controlled growth? *Why* is it controlling its growth? So that it can survive. Can there be some degree of intelligence here? There must be. What organism can regulate its growth up and down, based on an assessment of its current environment, adapt to ensure its survival, and not possess some degree of intelligence? These qualities set HIV apart from any other virus that we have ever previously encountered.

THE ANSWER: A COMBINATION OF NATURAL AND STANDARD MEDICAL THERAPIES

Due to the failure of all currently accepted standard medical therapies to completely halt the progress of HIV once a person is exposed, there exists a need for a more creative approach to its treatment. The goal of this approach should be to alter the stimuli that the virus receives from its intracellular environment so that it is encouraged to down-regulate its own growth and become dormant.

How do we accomplish this? Initially, we have tried to do it solely with drugs. Unfortunately, they have been shown to possess a high degree of toxicity and many side effects. HIV has also shown an ability to fight back if its environment becomes too inhospitable or toxic. It accomplishes this by mutating so that a specific drug no longer has the desired effect. This has occurred with AZT, and there is no reason to assume that it won't happen with any other antiviral medication.

Aside from drugs, another way to change the intracellular environment of your cells and strengthen your immune system is through the intake of certain natural substances. These include vitamins, herbs, and healthful foods. Just because a substance is natural in its origin does not diminish its ability to have a potent healing effect on the body. Natural substances can effectively stimulate the body to maintain the strong host immune response necessary to inhibit the growth of HIV. If considered individually, the benefits of natural therapies are usually mild. However, when several are combined, their benefits become significant.

Let me explain further. The immune system possesses an incredible degree of complexity and resilience. It is comprised of millions of lymphocytes, monocytes, T-cells, macrophages, and neutrophils that all communicate with each other through a vast array of biochemical messengers. All of these cells are influenced, in part, by the nutritional state of the body. Their functioning is enhanced by the presence of certain vitamins and natural compounds and depressed by deficiencies of the same. Furthermore, the ability of the immune system to function effectively is influenced by the brain and the neuroendocrine system. The level of the immune system's functioning can therefore be influenced, to some extent, by your thoughts, feelings, and emotions. By accessing the immune system through these channels, both nutritionally and psychologically, you can enhance its ability to remain strong.

Finally, when you *combine* a potent program of natural therapies with the appropriate amount of medication, you achieve the *ideal* treatment for HIV. This combination program creates a strong and balanced host immune response as well as a pharmacologic deterrent to the virus's replication. There are also fewer medication side effects because the drugs can be utilized at lower dosages.

The Comprehensive Healing Program for HIV is designed to combine both natural and standard medical therapies into a treatment program that can easily be integrated into the lifestyle of any HIV-positive individual. Its ability to promote a dormant viral state has become clear during the past five years of my practice experience and is supported by the study results and practice data that I will present to you later in this book.

DEFINING A DORMANT VIRAL STATE

Before we try to achieve a dormant viral state, we must first define in detail what we mean by this term. Shutting down HIV's ability to replicate itself allows us to prevent any further damage that it might cause to the immune system. There is a negative P-24 antigen test (indicating an absence of viral activity), no loss of T-cells (the cells most often destroyed by HIV), and an absence of symptoms. Achieving viral dormancy needs to be the top priority for the treatment of the HIV infection.

So how can you tell if the HIV infection has become dormant? First, you remain completely *asymptomatic*. As long as this situation continues, no matter how many T-cells you have, there is a significant degree of stability.

The second requirement for viral dormancy is to have a stable or increasing T-helper cell number. These cells protect you from what are commonly known as opportunistic infections. They are also the cells specifically targeted for infection by the HIV virus. (Please refer to the Lab Tests section of the Standard Medical Therapies chapter for a detailed discussion of the relevance of T-helper cells to HIV disease.)

Approximately three quarters of the patients who are following this program in its entirety experience either stable or increasing T-helper cell numbers in addition to remaining asymptomatic. If the Comprehensive Healing Program for HIV is begun early (greater than 300 T-helper cells per mm³), there is a high probability that you can arrest the progression of the HIV infection indefinitely and achieve viral dormancy. For example, *fewer than one out of ten patients who have come to see me with greater than 300 T-helper cells have progressed in their diagnosis during the past five years.* Additionally, thirty percent of the patients that I initially treated with symptomatic ARC (AIDS-related complex) have improved their condition and *reverted back* to their original asymptomatic status. These observations directly contradict the steadily declining course most often seen in patients who utilize standard medical therapies alone.

In some patients, the T-helper cell number has already fallen to very low levels. I know it is difficult for many of these patients not to be pessimistic about the future of their health. However, it is important to understand that your T-helper cell number *is not the entire picture of your immune system strength.* I have dozens of HIV-positive patients with T-helper cell numbers under two hundred who continue to remain stable and asymptomatic. This tells me that there are other components of the immune system that can be strengthened to help an HIV-positive individual remain healthy. If you can continue to strengthen these other aspects of the immune system, then a stable and asymptomatic level of health can be maintained.

Sometime in the near future, I am sure we will see medical advances to help us modulate the immune system and stimulate T-helper cell numbers to increase. If you can remain stable and asymptomatic long enough, then you will surely survive to benefit from these advances. The Comprehensive Healing Program for HIV can help you extend your lifetime in order to benefit from these new treatments as soon as they become available.

COMPREHENSIVE HEALING PROGRAM FOR HIV—A HISTORY

When I first attended the University of Texas Medical School in Houston, I was an idealistic young medical student who looked forward to learning how to best care for his patients. After my first year of training, however, I became disillusioned. I was being taught to view the human body predominantly through a microscope. I was shown how viruses, bacteria, and fungi could invade the human body and which drugs I should use to kill them. It was never explained to me *why* infections occurred in the first place or how to help keep a person from initially becoming sick.

This quickly frustrated me. I cared about preventing suffering, not just treating it once it had begun. As an undergraduate philosophy major I had been trained to seek the truth and investigate the underlying principles explaining why events occurred. My desire for knowledge was clearly not being satisfied.

I also felt, to some extent, that I was being brainwashed. Every morning at eight o'clock I would go into a huge, cavernous lecture hall and after five minutes the lights would go out and slides would begin to flash one after another in front of my eyes. The instructor would say something like, ". . . And the *Vibrio* organism causes cholera. Cholera is treated with high doses of trimethoprim-sulfamethoxizole. Typhoid can also cause the same symptoms but it is treated with chloramphenicol. The side effects of chloramphenicol include . . ." etc., etc., etc. This occurred during most of my first two years in medical school. There wasn't any discussion as to how the human body is designed to remain in a balanced state as long as it is properly cared for. In fact, there was almost no mention of many of the preventive concepts that I feel are the keys to maintaining good health. These include healthful nutrition, regular exercise, a positive attitude, and so on.

Because of my frustration, I ventured beyond standard medical training and began exploring the benefits of nutrition, herbs, vitamins, and other natural therapies. I acquired this knowledge from books, specialized courses, workshops, and practical experience. After several years of training, I felt competent to begin incorporating these techniques into a more complete and effective model of caring for my patients.

After graduating medical school in 1984, I came to San Francisco to do my internship in internal medicine at Kaiser Hospital. The treatment of AIDS was an integral part of my training as a medical intern. Since HIV was such a slowly progressive, chronic infection, I believed that there were a multitude of natural therapies that could be added to the standard medical regimen to help strengthen the immune system and prevent its breakdown. After a couple of additional years of experience in family practice and emergency medicine, I "hung out my shingle" and started practicing the kind of medicine that I believe in: the kind that combines the best of both natural and standard medical therapies.

My experience has been nothing short of amazing. From diabetes to HIV, many of my patients are able to feel better and decrease or completely eliminate their need for medication. They are happier and healthier and have higher-quality lives. I have learned that a combination approach, as opposed to one solely utilizing medications, is the next logical step in a comprehensive patient care model.

A PROGRAM BASED ON THEORY AND EXPERIENCE

The program of natural therapies that I initially developed for treating HIV included five categories: diet, vitamins, herbs, exercise, and stress reduction. It was my belief that if you worked very hard at these five categories, you would be able to maintain a healthy and strong immune system in spite of being HIV-positive. During the past five years I have learned that much more can be done to help keep HIV dormant. This includes providing a strong focus on emotional and spiritual growth as well as including standard medical therapies as an integral part of the treatment program. Therefore, based on this additional experience, the Comprehensive Healing Program for HIV now includes the following categories:

- **Natural therapies**
- **Psychological/emotional support**
- **Standard medical therapies**

It is extremely important to understand that the ability of this program to arrest the progression of the HIV infection is inherent in *the combined benefit* of all three categories. Each may be helpful to some extent, but when taken together, they exert a powerful healing effect on the human body and can encourage the occurrence of a dormant viral state for an extended period of time.

Thirty months ago, to test how this program might work, I set up a research study with ten asymptomatic HIV-positive gay men. This number was determined by the amount of funding I could gather to help support this research. The study sought to compare patients following the Comprehensive Healing Program for HIV with those utilizing standard medical therapies alone. During the thirty-month study period, the results have shown that the study group participants achieved a much greater degree of immune system stability and freedom from infections than the comparison groups. In fact, there were no deaths and only one serious infection in the Comprehensive Healing Program group during the entire study period. These results and the exact protocol are presented in more detail in the appendix.

Throughout most of 1989, based on the positive results I was observing, I tried to obtain additional funding to expand my study. I applied to several of the local, regional, and national AIDS research organizations. For whatever reason, most likely because I wasn't testing a single drug, these applications were denied. It soon became evident to me that I would best serve the people most in need of this vital information by publishing it in the form of a book and then resuming my search for the additional funding necessary to support a larger-scale study of this approach.

In the next chapter, the results I have had utilizing this program are presented. I am convinced that I see less disease progression, fewer infections, and, most importantly, fewer deaths than are commonly reported in the HIV-positive community. My patients also seem to enjoy a higher quality of life than many others in their community. They remain positive and hopeful and eventually feel that they "have a handle" on how to most effectively manage this condition. This feeling allows them to continue growing and enjoying other aspects of their lives to the greatest extent possible. The information contained in this book can help you, too, to share in these benefits.

PRIVATE PRACTICE DATA

Many of my colleagues are specialists in HIV care. The majority of them are exceptionally talented doctors. However, as we share stories and discuss individual cases, I clearly see that my patients do better at avoiding the progression of their disease.

Most of my colleagues' patients worsen not because the medical care they receive is in any way deficient. Their disease progresses because their lifestyles, dietary habits, and stress-reduction programs are insufficient to preserve their health in the face of their HIV positivity. Aggressive intervention with natural therapies *must* occur if one is to significantly alter the course of this infection and achieve stability.

When I describe individuals who do not follow the Comprehensive Healing Program for HIV as "not doing well," I mean that the course of their illness is filled with severe symptoms, chronic pain, and multiple hospitalizations. They commonly experience conditions such as abscesses, intractable diarrhea, severe abdominal pain, and massive infections, which are responsible for many days in the hospital and an inferior quality of life.

It is not necessary for this much suffering to occur with HIV. Preventing its progression entails identifying several specific changes that need to occur in your diet and lifestyle, and following through with them. It takes looking inside yourself and continuing to grow one step at a time. It means including those standard medical therapies that are necessary and appropriate for your program to remain effective. When these steps are followed, results are much improved. I can honestly say that *three quarters of the HIV-positive patients who have followed this program in its entirety, and who began the program with greater than 250 T-helper cells, have either stable or higher numbers now than when they began the program several years ago.* Since most HIV-positive patients normally experience a progressive decline in their T-helper cell number over time, this is clearly an unusual result.

I am certainly not saying that my patients never get sick. However, the majority of them stay well for extremely long periods of time. If they do become ill, they recover from their infections quickly and have long periods that are predominantly symptom-free.

In addition, many of my patients have had T-helper cell counts below 250 for the better part of five years and have remained relatively asymptomatic the entire time. Let me repeat that: *under 250 T-helper cells for the better part of five years and relatively asymptomatic the entire time.* The majority of these patients are able to avoid symptoms such as thrush, hairy leukoplakia, weight loss, dementia, fatigue, lymphadenopathy, and most types of opportunistic infections. And if they do become ill, it is usually of short duration and low intensity. Is this what you hear from your friends and coworkers with regard to HIV? Not usually. With fewer than 250 T-helper cells, they usually experience many symptoms and infections. Following the Comprehensive Healing Program for HIV enables my patients to avoid much of the pain and suffering that might otherwise be seen at this level of immune-system functioning. Of course, the optimal situation is to begin following the Comprehensive Healing Program for HIV early (T-helper cell number at least 300 cells per cubic millimeter of whole blood), and then to preserve or improve the strength of your immune system for many years to come.

My experience has shown me that it is definitely possible to change the course of this disease from one of suffering and a quick demise to one that includes an extended period of happiness, insight, and personal growth. The ability of many of my patients to accomplish this comes from a lot of hard work, self-exploration, and positive changes in their lifestyles. It is my strong belief that following my recommendations will have a beneficial effect on your survival.

PRACTICE DATA

The following statistics have been gleaned from my private practice files. The numbers represent those patients who have used me as their primary-care physician during a surveillance period of 4.25 years (March 1987 to June 1991). The average time I have cared for each patient is 1.47 years.

The surveillance group began with the following patient profile:

Asymptomatic HIV(+)	85
ARC	19
AIDS	30
Total patients	*134*

The group ended with the following patient profile:

Asymptomatic HIV(+)	85
ARC	10
AIDS	36
Deaths	3
Total patients	*134*

During the surveillance period of 4.25 years, the following events occurred:

Progression from asymptomatic HIV(+) to ARC	3 of 85	(4%)
Progression from asymptomatic HIV(+) to AIDS	3 of 85	(4%)
Progression from ARC to AIDS	6 of 19	(32%)
Reversal from ARC to asymptomatic HIV(+)	6 of 19	(32%)

AIDS patients who died	3 of 30	(10%)
Additional mortality (from categories other than AIDS)	None	(0%)
Patients who remained stable or improved their diagnosis	119 of 134	(89%)
Overall survival rate	131 of 134	(98%)

It should be noted that of the three deaths in my practice during this time, two were in patients who had active opportunistic infections and T-helper-cell counts of less than twenty when they first came to see me.

PROGRESSION REVERSALS

During the surveillance period, six patients *reversed their condition,* changing their diagnosis from ARC back to HIV-positive. That is, there were *reversals* in disease progression in one third of the ARC patients who came to see me during this period. The requirements for my definition of a diagnosis reversal include (1) a persistent rise in the T-helper cell number by at least 100 cells and (2) total elimination of any chronic symptoms, such as thrush, diarrhea, and weight loss, that were previously present. These patients made the appropriate changes in their diet, lifestyle, and medications, and achieved significant improvement in their conditions.

As many of you know, the usual course of HIV is one of a steady decline. That is why totally eliminating long-standing symptoms and increasing the T-helper cell number by at least 100 cells per mm^3 is such a *highly unusual* result. That these changes occurred in one third of the ARC patients who have followed my program is further proof of its ability to significantly alter the course of the HIV condition.

The natural history of HIV is usually reported as much more virulent than the course experienced by the majority of my patients. This is illustrated by a 1991 U.S. Department of Veterans Affairs study on HIV disease. In preliminary reports, the data from

NATURAL THERAPIES

Summary of Natural Therapy Recommendations

1. Diet
Immune Enhancement Diet (to follow)

2. Vitamins and Nutritional Supplements
AM (With Breakfast)

Kal Multi-Fours	2 tabs
Twinlab Vitamin C 1000mg	2 caps
Twinlab Vitamin E 400 IU	1 cap
Marine Carotene 25,000 IU	1 cap
Twinlab Allerdophilus	1 cap

PM (With Dinner)

Kal Multi-Fours	2 tabs
Twinlab Vitamin C 1000mg	2 caps
Twinlab Vitamin E 400 IU	1 cap
Twinlab Allerdophilus	1 cap

(continued)

3. **Herbs**
   RESIST: four capsules taken three times a day on an
   empty stomach (one-half hour before or two hours after
   meals) with plenty of water. Additional herbs as per
   chapter recommendations.
4. **Exercise**
   Aerobic exercise three to five times per week for at
   least thirty minutes per session.
5. **Stress Reduction**
   A fifteen- to twenty-minute period of deep relaxation
   (relaxation tape, meditation, or yoga) twice daily.

DIET

*"Let thy food be thy medicine, and thy
medicine be thy food"*

Hippocrates

"Eating" is an activity that we practice several times a day. Based
on the composition of each meal, different hormones are released
into the bloodstream. These hormones affect the way we feel and
how our bodies function. For us to feel good and possess abundant
energy, our diets need to be healthful.

There is no shortage of controversy when it comes to the
question of what constitutes a healthful diet. In this chapter, I will
present to you a diet that will strengthen and balance your immune
system. *It is important to understand that this diet constitutes the
central foundation of the Comprehensive Healing Program for HIV.* If
you follow its recommendations, every other part of the program
will work in an enhanced fashion.

I have tried to make this diet easy to integrate into an average person's lifestyle. You can go to your favorite restaurant, attend your best friend's dinner parties and continue to feel that you are a valid, participating member of society. You can remain within the healthful boundaries of this program and continue to enjoy every moment of your life.

So what constitutes a healthy diet? First, your food must be *natural and minimally processed.* This allows your body to absorb and process the correct concentration of nutrients. It also prevents the body from being exposed to artificial chemicals that may negatively affect its functioning. Second, because the body has unusually high metabolic needs in the presence of an HIV infection, your diet must contain an *abundance* of vitamins, minerals, calories and protein. Meeting these requirements will help support and strengthen your immune system in the long term.

A less concrete reason for eating a healthful, well-balanced diet, is that it can be another way to show your body that you care for it, love it, and are willing to do everything in your power to support it. When your body is convinced that you truly care, when it senses your nurturing and love, your immune system becomes strengthened.

The Immune Enhancement Diet— General Principles

1. Increase your consumption of *whole grains* (brown rice, oats, cracked wheat, barley, corn, rye, millet, quinoa, and buckwheat). Always prepare more than you need. You can keep the leftovers in the refrigerator for a week. Add them to soups and other dishes. Attempt to have a portion of cooked whole grains *at least* once a day.

2. Increase your consumption of *vegetables* (fresh, steamed, or stir-fried). Eat as many of them as you can. They provide plentiful amounts of fiber, vitamins, and minerals.

3. Increase your consumption of *fresh fruit.* Use fruits as snacks and as a natural pick-me-up instead of processed sugar products.

4. Increase your consumption of *natural soups, teas,* and *warm beverages.* Optimal beverages include water, herb teas, fruit juices, and roasted-grain coffee substitutes such as Inka, Cafix, and Postum. These are nutritious beverages, as opposed to sugar-laden soft drinks. Mineral water, such as Calistoga or Perrier is fine. Do not drink anything that is *ice* cold. Your body will have to expend energy to warm it up. This depletes energy that could otherwise be utilized by your immune system. Quick, inexpensive, and extremely nutritious soups are found in the many varieties of Westbrae Ramen, and Nile Spice instant soups which can be found in most health-food stores.

5. *Eat a nutritious breakfast* every day. Hot whole-grain cereals are an important part of an optimal breakfast. High-fiber breads, toast, and cold cereals made from whole grains are the next best choice Healthful breads include Alvarado St. Bakery, Orowheat, and others that are made from whole grains and are high in fiber and low in additives and sugar. A high-quality breakfast provides strength and good nutrition at the very beginning of the day. Include a cup of hot herb tea or roasted-grain beverage with your morning meal to help promote efficient digestion.

6. Eat plenty of *onions, garlic,* and *ginger.*

7. The best oils to use are high-quality *olive* and *sesame.*

8. Eat *locally grown, seasonal foods*—organic, if possible.

9. Make sure that your diet provides you with an adequate amount of protein (see p. 25). Recommended protein sources include fish, poultry, legumes, soy products, whole grains, and an occasional portion of red meat.

10. *Limit your dairy consumption* to five percent of your total diet. Most people have a limited tolerance for dairy products (milk, butter, cheese, yogurt, etc.) that when exceeded can cause the production of excess gas, loose bowel movements, and even fatigue. This situation is not optimal for the efficient functioning of your digestive system. If dairy products are limited to approximately five percent of your total dietary volume, you will usually not experience any of these symptoms.

11. *Avoid sugar, alcohol, and caffeine.*

12. *Avoid raw foods* such as clams, oysters, marinated (uncooked) fish, sushi, very rare meats, and undercooked eggs. These can contain infectious bacteria and intestinal parasites.

13. *Combine and balance foods properly.* Do not eat vegetables and fruits at the same time. When eaten together, they promote inefficient digestion due to the different enzymes and digestive time that each requires. Grains and either vegetables or beans, combined with a small amount of a dairy product and herb tea is the optimal combination of foods. Eat more grains and vegetables than fruits to keep your diet alkaline. Rest for *at least* ten minutes after each meal to promote healthful digestion.

Energy Levels of Various Foods

The following list assigns foods to different energy levels. Energy level 1 represents foods that are medicinal in their healing properties.

Energy Level 1

UNLIMITED QUANTITIES ARE ENCOURAGED—AT LEAST 60 PERCENT OF YOUR DIET.

carrots	raw garlic	avocados
sprouts	shitake mushrooms	bananas
broccoli	brown rice	apples
cabbage	barley	oranges
spinach	oatmeal	strawberries
vegetarian soups	lentils	berries
sunflower seeds	bulgar wheat	grapes
almonds	shoyu (aged soy sauce)	raisins
beans	ginger	

Other lightly steamed or stir-fried vegetables, including red cabbage, celery, red chard, Swiss chard, cauliflower, beets, onions, etc.

Energy Level 2

UNLIMITED QUANTITIES—AT LEAST 20 PERCENT OF YOUR DIET.

vegetable juices	yogurt	eggs
fruit juices*	potatoes	peanuts
whole-grain breads	yams	corn
sprouted-seed breads	papayas	cashews
whole-grain pastas	lemon	olive oil
nut butters	herb teas	spring water

*Fruit juice is best diluted with an equal amount of water due to its high acid content.

Energy Level 3

SUPPLEMENTS.

Supplements are used to enhance the diet. They are not meant to replace a healthful selection of foods. Please refer to the section on nutritional supplements for more information regarding their appropriate selection and usage.

Energy Level 4

CONSUMPTION OF THESE FOODS OR SUBSTANCES SHOULD BE KEPT TO A MINIMUM.

coffee	desserts	ice cream
honey	dry cereals	cookies

Energy Level 5

THESE FOODS OR SUBSTANCES ARE BEST COMPLETELY AVOIDED.

smoked meats	alcohol	white sugar
canned vegetables	drugs	white flour
TV dinners	preservatives	chocolate
cigarettes	sulfur dioxide	raw fish and meats

Breakfast

Breakfast is the most important meal of the day. In the morning, most people immediately begin expending energy at a high rate. We leave for work, perform errands, and quickly begin to face the day's many stresses. Accordingly, it is important that we provide our bodies with high-quality fuel right from the start. If a person skips breakfast or just has a quick cup of coffee, he has not provided his body with adequate fuel to start the day.

Your immune system is the most sensitive system of your body to your energy level. When you are stressed, your heart beats faster and your muscles work harder. Your mind becomes stimulated and adrenaline is released into your bloodstream. Energy is diverted away from your immune system and used for other bodily functions. Eating breakfast ensures that there is an abundance of energy at the very beginning of the day to help prevent negative physiologic effects that might occur if you become stressed.

The ideal breakfast contains protein, fiber, carbohydrates, and fat. The protein and fat can come from eggs, whole grains, milk, nuts, and/or yogurt. Protein supplies the building blocks for cell regeneration and repair. Carbohydrates are best found in hot whole-grain cereals, granola, whole-grain pancakes, waffles, toast, and fruit. High-fiber foods provide a matrix in which the other nutrients can be healthfully digested. They improve the circulation to the digestive system. It is also helpful to have a warm drink in the morning to help "stoke your fire" and get the digestive processes going after a long night's sleep (consumption of caffeine is *not* necessary).

Protein

For the immune system to remain strong, it is extremely important to consume an adequate amount of protein. Inadequate protein intake results in lowered resistance to infection, poor wound healing, weight loss, and a general lack of vigor. If you do not consume adequate protein, the immune system will gradually weaken over time.

The recommended amount of protein for an individual who is under a "moderate" amount of stress is 0.4 grams per pound. A 170-pound individual would therefore require an intake of 68 grams of protein per day. Below you will find a table that lists many common foods and the amount of protein they contain. Estimate your daily protein intake. If you are not getting the recommended amount of protein for your weight, find the foods on the table that provide a large amount of protein, such as fish, chicken, soy products, cheese, beans, seeds, and nuts, and increase them in your diet.

The debate about the benefits of vegetable protein over animal protein is a long standing one and will surely not be settled here. My feeling is that it probably has more relevance to cardiovascular health than immune system strength. The most important points I am trying to convey are that your protein consumption should be varied in nature, of adequate quantity, and combined with appropriate amounts of other healthful foods in your diet such as whole grains, fresh vegetables, fruits, and so on.

Protein consumption can also be supplemented. Protein supplements can be taken as powder, liquids, tablets, or snack bars. Bear Valley Meal Pack bars can be found in most health food stores and provide 16 grams of protein per bar. Gainer's Fuel and Amino Fuel, both made by TwinLab Inc., provide 15 grams of protein per serving. The best source for your protein and other nutrients, however, is from a healthful and balanced diet.

Vegetables

You cannot eat too many vegetables. They provide your body with large amounts of vitamins, minerals, and fibers. Raw, steamed, or stir-fried, they are among nature's most nutritious and healthful foods. They are especially healthful when added to soups so that the nutrients contained within the cells can dissolve into a warm and easily digestible broth. The absorption of nutrients from soups requires virtually no expenditure of digestive energy and, therefore, is an optimal way to obtain beneficial nutrition.

Protein Sources*

(Minimum requirement: 0.4 grams per pound of body weight)

SOURCE	QUAN-TITY	PRO-TEIN	SOURCE	QUAN-TITY	PRO-TEIN
Meat			**Dairy**		
liver	4 oz	30 g	cottage cheese		
hamburger	4 oz	25 g	creamed	1 cup	31 g
steak	4 oz	25 g	uncreamed	1 cup	44 g
lamb	4 oz	20 g	cheese		
chicken	4 oz	20 g	cheddar	4 oz	28 g
fish	4 oz	25 g	swiss	4 oz	28 g
			milk	1 cup	8 g
Vegetarian			yogurt	1 cup	8 g
tofu	4 oz	10 g	egg	1	7 g
red beans	1 cup	14 g			
soybeans	1 cup	14 g	**Grains**		
chickpeas	1 cup	41 g	most grains	1 cup	3–5 g
lentils	1 cup	16 g	brown rice	1 cup	5 g
black beans	1 cup	12 g	white rice	1 cup	5 g
alfalfa sprouts	1 cup	5 g	oatmeal	1 cup	5 g
green beans	1 cup	2 g	bread	1 slice	2 g
potato (baked)	1	4 g			
			Seeds		
Nuts			sesame	1 cup	42 g
peanuts	1 cup	60 g	sunflower	1 cup	24 g
almonds	1 cup	25 g			
cashews	1 cup	15 g			

*All quantities are of cooked foods.

Whole Grains

A lack of whole grains is one of the biggest deficiencies in the standard American diet. Whole grains provide fiber, vitamins, and trace minerals that are extremely important to keep the immune system healthy. For years, large food producers tried to convince us that their bleached-white-flour products were as healthful as those made from whole-grain flour. Remember how the Wonder Bread television commercial stated that it contained all of the vitamins and minerals necessary to build strong bones and healthy bodies? White bread has such minimal fiber that it indirectly contributes to heart disease and colon cancer by replacing other foods in the diet that contain higher amounts of fiber. Only in the past few years has fiber become enough of a health issue that we are adding whole grains back into our diets in adequate amounts.

Fiber confers an important health benefit by stimulating the immune-enhancing cells called Peyer's patches found in the lining of the intestines. When stimulated, these cells help activate and strengthen the immune system by producing antibodies, which are the body's first line of defense against disease in the intestinal tract. Whole grains provide large amounts of fiber that stimulate the blood flow to these cells, thus enhancing their ability to function.

Another reason that fiber is so healthful is that it helps cleanse the colon of toxins, such as fats and bile acids, by absorbing them and removing them from the body. Fats and bile acids have been shown to promote cancer. Abundant fiber also helps to prevent parasites and other intestinal infections.

I would like to make one additional point with regard to whole grains and fiber. There is an important distinction between the consumption of flour products made from whole grains and the consumption of the *intact whole grain itself.* Intact whole grains such as oats, brown rice, cracked wheat, barley, corn, rye, quinoa, millet, and buckwheat have a strengthening effect on the digestive system. *The consumption of flour products is not equivalent.* The digestion of the intact whole grain gives the entire digestive system a toning workout. If you were trying to strengthen your muscles, you wouldn't give them a workout with two-pound weights. You would progressively increase your workout to keep your muscles strong. That is why *intact* whole grains are so strengthening to the digestive system.

One of the simplest ways to consume an adequate amount of intact whole grains is to cook several days' worth and store the leftovers in the refrigerator. Just combine a portion of the refrigerated whole grains with a small amount of simmering water or place them in the microwave for two minutes to reheat. You can then eat them as a hot cereal or side dish. They can also be added to soups, stir-fry, or other dishes quickly and easily. You'll find several basic recipes for the preparation of whole grains (and a recipe for an extremely healthful broth called "immunity soup") at the end of this chapter.

Fruit

In general, fruit is an extremely healthful addition to your diet. Most fruits are high in vitamins, minerals, and fiber and are a healthful source of natural sweetness.

A frequently asked question is whether individuals who are trying to rebuild their immune systems should consume only organic produce. A recent study performed by researchers at Rutgers University showed that organic produce was, on the average, 87 percent higher in minerals than nonorganic produce. Calcium, magnesium, potassium, manganese, iron, and copper were all found to be markedly higher in the organic produce. Mineral content is higher because commercial produce is usually grown in weaker, less nutritious soil.

While organic produce has been shown to have greater quantities of vitamins and minerals, it is also more expensive and sometimes difficult to obtain. Consider organic produce to be superior in its health benefits to nonorganic produce, and use it whenever possible. However, it is not "required" for your healing program to be successful.

Make sure that you wash your produce with plenty of water. If there is a noticeable residue, use a small amount of mild dishwashing detergent. (I am not in favor of washing fruits and vegetables in dilute chlorine bleach as some people recommend.) Even if your produce is organic, it is important to wash it thoroughly. Microorganisms from the soil can be a source of infection, such as mycobacteria, several fungal diseases, and intestinal parasites, in individuals who are immunocompromised.

Fruit contains a high concentration of natural sugar. Many HIV-positive individuals have noticed that even the sugar from fruit and fruit juice is enough to cause them to develop an overgrowth of thrush, a common oral infection in HIV-positive individuals caused by the yeast *Candida albicans*. As with anything that you eat, its effect on you depends upon the quantity consumed. Too much fruit on a daily basis can cause thrush to become exacerbated or even appear for the first time. If you have any difficulty with thrush, processed sugar should be the first thing that you eliminate from your diet. If the problem continues, fruit and fruit juice should be eliminated as the next step. (Refer to the section entitled Treatment of Specific Conditions and Symptoms for more information on how to prevent and eliminate thrush.)

During the past five years, it has been my experience that most individuals who are following the dietary recommendations of the Comprehensive Healing Program for HIV can eat fruit in unlimited quantities without developing thrush because they avoid consuming excessive amounts of the three substances discussed below.

The Negatives: Sugar, Caffeine, and Alcohol

The negative dietary habits that cause the most problems to the immune system are the excessive consumption of sugar, caffeine, and alcohol. These three items, especially if combined with skipping breakfast and an inadequate protein intake, will quickly weaken the immune system.

Sugar and the Immune System

Since 1973 there have been several scientific studies that have provided strong evidence of sugar's negative effect on the immune system's ability to function effectively. White blood cells, including T-helper cells, are adversely affected by excessive amounts of sugar in the bloodstream. A research study published in the *American Journal of Clinical Nutrition* in 1973 showed that when white blood cells were exposed to high levels of sugar in the bloodstream, they had a decreased ability to engulf bacteria (phagocytosis). The greatest effect occurred between one and two hours after a liquid sugar meal, but *their ability was depressed for up to five hours afterwards.*

In this study, test subjects were divided into five groups. Group 1 received a placebo and acted as the control for the study. Groups 2, 3, 4, and 5 received a liquid drink containing 6, 12, 18, and 24 teaspoons of sugar, respectively. Blood samples were taken from these individuals at ½, 1, 2, 3, and 5 hours after consuming the drink. The samples were then incubated with a suspension of staphylococcus bacteria and were viewed under a microscope. The number of bacteria that were engulfed by each white blood cell was counted and averaged for each group.

The results of the study showed that the group which consumed no sugar had an average of 14 bacteria engulfed by each white blood cell. There was a progressive decline in the number of bacteria engulfed by each group's white cells as their sugar consumption increased. At 6 teaspoons of sugar, the average number of engulfed bacteria was 10 per white blood cell, at 12 teaspoons of sugar the average number was 5.5 per white blood cell, at 18 teaspoons the average was 2 per white blood cell, and after 24 teaspoons of sugar, the average number of bacteria destroyed per white blood cell was only 1. Ingesting 24 teaspoons of sugar (the equivalent of two cans of soda) produced a 92 percent decrease in the white blood cell's ability to engulf bacteria.

Other studies performed at Rockefeller University in New York provide evidence that protein molecules, which are present in all cells, can be adversely affected by elevated levels of sugar in the bloodstream. High concentrations of sugar combine with protein molecules to form advanced glycosylation end products, or AGE's. AGE particles act like glue, binding protein molecules together to form a rigid lattice network known as cross-linking. These large protein molecules can inhibit the functioning of the immune system, blur vision, and cause damage to the kidneys and lungs.

Ingesting large amounts of processed sugar also puts great stress on the body in general. The total sugar content normally present in your bloodstream is approximately one teaspoon. When a person consumes a can of soda or a bowl of ice cream (containing an average sugar content of *twelve teaspoons*), the digestive system must work extremely hard to prevent this amount of sugar from entering the bloodstream all at once. To produce sufficient insulin for processing this amount of sugar, the pancreas must also work extremely hard. This stress is not healthful for your immune system.

Sugar can also act like a drug. As you *decrease* the amount you consume, you may experience withdrawal symptoms including headaches, irritability, nausea, and anxiety. If these occur, it is best to completely eliminate processed sugar from your diet in "cold turkey" fashion. The symptoms will last for a few days and then you will begin to feel much better. Drink lots of clear fluids, such as water and herb teas, take plenty of B-complex vitamins (50 milligrams three times per day) and vitamin C (2 grams three times per day) and eat filling, nutritious meals consisting of whole grains and vegetables. You can also eat a small amount of fruit if you feel poorly. This is the best way to eliminate, or greatly diminish, your cravings for sugar.

Once you are free from sugar, you will notice that you feel calmer and more relaxed. Your thinking becomes clearer. Your stress level becomes lower and you will begin to feel much more connected to your body. Awareness of your body allows you to be more in touch with its needs. Also, your energy level will improve. This increase in energy can now be utilized by your immune system.

If your diet is basically natural and wholesome and includes a healthful amount of whole grains, fruits and vegetables, and so on, a small amount of processed sugar will not adversely affect your immune system. One to three times a week, a small amount of processed sugar is allowable under the Comprehensive Healing Program for HIV.

Advertising Tricks

It is *imperative* that you read labels. On every package of food that has been processed, you should check the label for sugar and other sweeteners. Ingredients are listed on food labels in order of greater to lesser weight. It is important to understand that the ingredients listed fourth, fifth, and sixth may, when added together, outweigh the ingredient listed first.

Sugar equivalents can be listed under many different names. Corn syrup, dextrose, maltose, sucrose, glucose, and fructose are all highly concentrated sweeteners with the same negative effect on the immune system. If several of these are present, the cumulative amount of sugar makes the product unhealthful. *If only one ingredient is present and it is not among the first three on the label,* the product is safe to consume.

Since the consumption of sugar is so prevalent in our society (average consumption: 128 pounds per person per year or 1 pound per person every three days), I am frequently asked what sources of sugar *are* acceptable. The most healthful way to sweeten your food is by adding fruit to it. Foods that are sweetened with fruit juice are also acceptable. Small amounts of honey, pure maple syrup, and molasses can also be used as sweeteners. Keep in mind that the goal is to avoid *an unnaturally high concentration* of sugar. When you use fruit or fruit juice as a sweetener, you are providing your body with a natural concentration of sugar that it is able to process without causing stress to your system.

The following graph summarizes the best and worse choices for sweet foods.

Caffeine

A recent editorial in the British Medical Journal called caffeine "the world's most popular drug." The average American drinks approximately 32 gallons of caffeinated soft drinks and 28 gallons of coffee a year. This adds up to a total of 60 gallons of caffeinated drinks a year!

Healing occurs when the body is relaxed and its energy can be channeled inward. Consuming caffeine regularly impedes the body's ability to heal because caffeine blocks the cells' ability to regenerate its energy resources. No wonder you need a second and third cup of coffee to keep you going after the first one wears off!

When my wife stopped drinking coffee she was amazed at the *increase* in her energy level, instead of the decrease she had expected. This occurred because her body could go through the entire day at its own healthful pace. Her energy was conserved and balanced.

Decaffeinated coffee is not as detrimental to the healing process as caffeinated coffee. However, it is not a healthful beverage, either. It contains many of the chemicals and acids found in caffeinated coffee. Instead of coffee, there are several healthful alternatives that may be consumed in the morning to help you get a good start on the day. These include tasty and nutritious roasted-whole-grain coffee substitutes such as Inka, Cafix, and Postum. Additionally, there are a variety of herb teas that you can drink to help provide you with an acceptable alternative to coffee.

A moderate intake of caffeine (one cup of strong coffee), up to three times per week, is allowable as part of the Comprehensive Healing Program for HIV.

Alcohol

When consumed in excess, alcohol is a poison to every system of your body. It depresses the nervous system, inhibits the bone marrow's ability to regenerate blood cells, depletes B vitamins, and is dehydrating.

If you are HIV-positive, alcohol is best consumed in very small quantities or avoided altogether. Many individuals following the Comprehensive Healing Program for HIV have decided to avoid alcohol completely and are happy about their decision. They view it as another positive growth step that HIV has brought about in their lives.

The maximum amount of alcohol recommended by the Comprehensive Healing Program for HIV is three glasses of wine or beer per week. Avoid hard liquor entirely because of its higher concentration of alcohol. It is a good idea to drink lots of water before and after drinking alcohol to dilute it and replace the fluids lost due to its dehydrating effect.

Positive Motivation

The process of eating a healthful, natural diet requires two things: (1) *desire* and (2) *awareness,* the ability to see through slick marketing claims and identify exactly what makes up the products that you are eating.

Another ingredient for success when it comes to improving your diet is willingness to establish new habits and rituals. A patient of mine pointed out that it wasn't a cup of fresh-brewed coffee in the morning that he missed. It was the "ritual" of waking up to a hot, fresh-brewed beverage that helped him awaken his senses after sleep. He now substitutes a freshly brewed pot of herb tea or roasted-grain coffee as his morning ritual and is satisfied.

Allow yourself to begin incorporating some of the changes that I have outlined in this chapter on a daily basis. Start small. Eat breakfast every day. Begin avoiding caffeine, sugar, and alcohol. Drink plenty of water. Buy some herb teas and find a favorite. These are some easy, healthful changes to begin with. Next, eat more fruits and vegetables. Make sure your protein intake is adequate. Eat less junk food. All of these will help, and after a few weeks of combining these changes together into a program of healthful eating, you will begin to feel the difference! You will have more energy and feel stronger. You may also begin feeling better about yourself. Your diet is the place to start. A healthful diet is the foundation of any healing program. Now is the time to start yours!

Healthful Recipes

BROWN RICE — BASIC RECIPE

1 cup brown rice
2¼ cups water
1 clove garlic
dash of salt or shoyu (soy sauce)

Rinse rice in a large strainer. Place in a large covered saucepan with water, salt or shoyu, and garlic. Bring to a rolling boil. Turn down to simmer. Cook 40 to 50 minutes (until water has boiled off).*

BARLEY AND RICE

1 cup brown rice
⅓ cup barley
3½ cup water
dash of salt

Mix ingredients together and cook one hour on low flame after bringing to a rolling boil. A healthful nutty combination of grains results.*

ORIGINAL OATMEAL

⅓ cup oats
1 cup water
dash of salt

Stir oats into briskly boiling salted water. Reduce flame and cook for 5 minutes or until water is absorbed. In order to enhance and sweeten the flavor of the oats, you may add raisins or sliced bananas, apples, or peaches and, if desired, a *small* amount of honey. A dash of milk may also be added.

CRACKED WHEAT CEREAL

1 cup cracked or bulgur wheat
2 cups water
dash of salt

Flavor-enhancing variations: Add one or all of the following ingredients prior to heating: ½ teaspoon grated ginger, 1 clove minced garlic, a vegetable bouillon cube, a small amount of shoyu (soy sauce), sliced carrots, and *shiitake* mushrooms.

Heat the ingredients to a rolling boil. Cover and reduce heat to simmer. Cook for 20 to 30 minutes or until water is absorbed. (Bulgur cooks for 20 minutes, while cracked wheat takes 30 minutes.) Add sliced bananas, sliced almonds, raisins, a small amount of honey or molasses, or a dash of milk and cinnamon for added flavor and sweetness.

BARLEY-CABBAGE CASSEROLE

1 cup barley
2 cups water
½ teaspoon salt
2 tablespoons sesame oil
½ cabbage
shoyu (soy sauce) to taste
bread crumbs

Wash and drain barley. Add water and salt and cook covered for approximately 45 minutes. Add cooked barley to the cabbage, which has been chopped small and sauteed in sesame oil. Mix, season with salt, and add shoyu. Place in a casserole dish, sprinkle with bread crumbs, and bake in a preheated oven at 350 degrees. Cook approximately 20 minutes or until golden brown.

IMMUNITY SOUP

Soak:
6 *shiitake* mushrooms in 2 cups of
    water for 20 minutes.

Chop the mushrooms (discard
stems).

Add:
chopped mushrooms and soaking
    water to 4 cups of spring water in
    saucepan. Bring to a boil.

Simmer 10 minutes.

Add:
2 carrots, thinly sliced
2 stalks celery, thinly sliced
1 onion, diced
2 cloves garlic, minced
other chopped vegetables as desired.

Simmer 15 minutes.

Add:
1-inch piece of white daikon radish, diced
1 small bunch chopped parsley
⅓ cup wakame sea vegetable, chopped and soaked for 15 minutes (discard water)
a pinch of thyme
¼ pound tofu, cut into small pieces

Simmer 15 minutes.

Add:
½ to 1 cup *cooked* brown rice
3 tablespoons miso (mixed with some water into a paste)

Flavor with salt, pepper, and/or shoyu to taste.

Simmer 5 minutes (do not boil). . . .
Enjoy!
(Many thanks to nutritionist Elizabeth Huntley, Ph.D., for this recipe.)

VITAMINS AND NUTRITIONAL SUPPLEMENTS

There is an increasing amount of scientific evidence to support the use of vitamin supplements for both the prevention and treatment of disease. In spite of this, the medical establishment still discourages anything but their most minimal use. In this section, I hope to present data to support the use of vitamins and other nutritional supplements as an effective way to strengthen the immune system.

Although good nutrition is best obtained from your food, sometimes our diets are less than optimal. In a conversation with Dr. Howard Riddick, a researcher for the U.S. Department of Agriculture, it was confirmed that none of the 21,500 Americans surveyed during the most recently published USDA National Food Consumption Study (1984) consumed 100 percent of the RDA (Recommended Dietary Allowances) for the following combination of vitamins and minerals: Vitamins A, B_1, B_2, B_6, B_{12}, and C; calcium; and iron.

Additionally, it is well recognized that malnutrition plays an important role in the course and outcome of AIDS. Dr. Charles Halsted, chief of the internal medicine department at the University of California at Davis Medical School, found that AIDS attacks the intestinal cells that absorb vital nutrients *during the early stages of the disease.* He went on to state that "poor absorption of nutrients can be one of the early causes of malnutrition in patients."

The goal of this part of the Comprehensive Healing Program for HIV is to ensure that the body is provided with the nutrients necessary for the immune system to function optimally 100 percent of the time.

The government's RDAs (see fig. 1) were initially arrived at by depriving army trainees of a single nutrient until they began to manifest symptoms of a deficiency disease. These diseases include rickets (vitamin D), beriberi (vitamin B_1), scurvy (vitamin C), and pernicious anemia (vitamin B_{12}). When these diseases occur, after months of absent or minimal intake, they constitute a total breakdown of many of the body's major systems including the skin, blood, and nervous system. The RDAs were established by the U.S. government as an arbitrarily "safe" margin above the level at which vitamin deficiency diseases occur. Although these levels prevent deficiency diseases from occurring, they are not designed to promote *peak performance* of the body. In addition, they are for the benefit of the general population and should not be considered adequate for individuals faced with the special circumstance of illness or stress. Applying the RDAs to an HIV-positive individual is like taking a high-performance race car, in the middle of a grueling race, and giving it just enough octane in its fuel to keep it from breaking down. It may finish the race but it is certainly not going to win.

The following are three additional reasons why individuals who are HIV-positive or otherwise have depressed immune systems, can benefit from taking vitamins and other nutritional supplements:

1. Vitamins and minerals are sensitive compounds that break down easily when food is cooked, exposed to light, or stored for long periods of time. Vitamins can also break down when food is handled roughly or processed. Much of the food that makes its way into urban supermarkets has been picked before it is ripe, transported long distances, and treated with waxes, fumigants, and other chemicals to preserve its flavor and appearance. Do you think this is the quality of food that nature originally intended for us to eat?

2. Additionally, the soil in which most of our food is grown has been overworked by the widespread use of petrochemical fertilizers. No longer do farmers allow their fields to lie fallow for one year out of every three to rest and regenerate. Overworking the soil depletes it of essential nutrients and minerals that are necessary for the immune system to function effectively.

3. Modern living is stressful to our bodies. There is extensive pollution throughout our environment. The interaction of these pollutants with our cells can produce unhealthful byproducts known as free radicals. Free radicals are toxic to our

cells and produce unhealthful changes that can weaken the immune system and promote cancer. Antioxidant compounds, such as vitamins A, E, and C, beta carotene, selenium, and zinc, circulate throughout the body and help to neutralize toxic free radicals.

It is generally agreed that nutritional deficiencies have a negative effect on the functioning of the immune system. However, there continues to be increasing evidence that supplements can *enhance* the functioning of the immune system above the level that exists when no supplementation is provided.

In a 1986 study, published in the journal *Contemporary Nutrition,* the functioning of both T and B lymphocytes was enhanced by supplementary doses of vitamin A. Another controlled study published in *Immunology Letters* in 1985 showed that after one week of beta-carotene supplementation, normal volunteers had an increase in their T-helper cell number while their T-suppressor cell number remained the same.

The goal of the vitamin and nutritional supplement part of the Comprehensive Healing Program for HIV is to enhance the functioning of the immune system with the safe use of vitamins and other nutritional supplements.

The following is the recommended supplement program of the Comprehensive Healing Program for HIV:

Supplement Schedule

AM (With Breakfast)

KAL Multi-Fours	2 tabs
Twinlab Vitamin C 1000 mg	2 caps
Twinlab Vitamin E 400 IU	1 cap
Twinlab Marine Carotene 25,000 IU	1 cap
Twinlab Allerdophilus	1 cap

(continued)

PM (With Dinner)

KAL Multi-Fours	2 tabs
Twinlab Vitamin C 1000 mg	2 caps
Twinlab Vitamin E 400 IU	1 cap
Twinlab Allerdophilus	1 cap

The brands KAL and Twinlab are specifically recommended because of their extremely high quality, moderate cost, and widespread availability. These are also the specific products tested in the Comprehensive Healing Program for HIV Research Study. If these are unavailable, other brands may be substituted for the individual vitamins (C, E, and beta-carotene). However, I feel strongly that the KAL Multi-Fours and Twinlab Allerdophilus are a level above most generic brands when it comes to quality and efficacy.

The above regimen achieves the following objectives: (1) It provides the immune-compromised individual with an adequate dosage of all necessary vitamins and minerals. (2) It contains therapeutic amounts of antioxidants (vitamin C, vitamin E and beta-carotene). (3) It is easily tolerated by most individuals. (4) It is of minimal cost (approximately $25 per month).

As you can see from Figure 2, KAL Multi-Fours is the multivitamin-and-mineral supplement that is the foundation of this program. It is an all-purpose supplement that is blended together in an extremely gentle therapeutic herbal base. It is high in quality and well tolerated.

If low energy or fatigue is present, I often recommend substituting a multivitamin-and-mineral supplement with a higher dosage of B vitamins than the Multi-Fours. The substitute that I have had excellent results with is KAL's Mega-Vitamin. It contains a 75 milligram B complex and is in time-release form, so it can be taken once daily. For general use, however, I still prefer the Multi-Fours.

The next three vitamins on the supplement schedule are vitamin C, E, and Marine (beta) Carotene. These three vitamins are all antioxidants and have been shown in numerous studies to have a beneficial effect on the functioning of the immune system *when taken in therapeutic dosages.* Therapeutic dosages are defined as dosages above those recommended by the government's RDA. Acidophilus bacteria, in a highly potent and easily tolerated form (Twinlab Allerdophilus), completes the program.

The following additional information and research studies substantiate the use of these specific vitamins and nutritional supplements as part of a program to strengthen a weakened immune system.

Vitamin C

Since 1970, when he first recommended large doses of vitamin C to treat viral diseases such as influenza and some forms of cancer, two-time Nobel Prize winner Linus Pauling has been strongly criticized by members of the medical establishment for his views. Even though Dr. Pauling has amassed an enormous amount of data illustrating the benefits of Vitamin C for the treatment of these conditions, the people who control the money used for medical research continue to refuse to fund his grants. Hopefully, the current bias against the study of nutritional therapies to help the body fight disease will change as more positive results are published in the scientific literature.

Michael Castleman, in his book *Cold Cures,* reviewed the current medical literature on vitamin C and noted some interesting findings. Since 1945, thirty-one studies have tested vitamin C against the common cold. Fifteen showed no effect. Sixteen showed significant benefit described as a 30 to 50 percent decrease in the severity and duration of symptoms. Why such different outcomes from these studies?

Upon closer inspection, the fifteen studies that showed no effect from supplementing with this vitamin all used low doses of vitamin C (250 milligrams or less) for short periods of time. All sixteen studies that showed a significant benefit from vitamin C supplementation used high dosages (2,000 milligrams or greater) and provided the vitamin from the moment any symptoms appeared until they completely resolved. It appears that there is a threshold level above which vitamin C boosts the immune system against viral infections. Since HIV is a chronic viral infection, there is good reason to believe that the same immune-stimulating effect that vitamin C has against viral influenza might be of benefit in helping to combat HIV.

Steve Harakeh, Raxit Jariwalla, and Dr. Pauling published a study in the *Proceeds of the National Academy of Sciences* in 1990 entitled "Suppression of Human Immunodeficiency Virus Replication by Ascorbate in Chronically and Acutely Infected Cells." The results showed that continuous exposure of HIV-infected cells to nontoxic ascorbate concentrations (vitamin C) resulted in significant inhibition of both total virus and P-24 antigen formation. The ascorbate, in these concentrations, did not adversely affect either the host cell's metabolic activity or its rate of protein synthesis. Reverse transcriptase, the enzyme inhibited by AZT, showed a three- to fourteen-fold decrease in activity when exposed to high concentrations of ascorbate.

This study provides evidence that vitamin C directly inhibits the growth and replication of HIV. Additional studies need to be performed in humans to look at its effect on such indicators as freedom from opportunistic infections, growth of viral cultures, and T-cell subset numbers. Hopefully, funding for additional studies will follow these positive preliminary results.

Vitamin C is extremely helpful to the immune system in other ways. These include enhanced proliferation of T cells, increased levels of circulating IgA, IgM, and IgG antibodies, and improvement in the ability of white blood cells to engulf bacteria (phagocytosis). In fact, the intracellular concentration of vitamin C in the white blood cell (lymphocytes specifically), has been shown to be greater than ten times that in most other cells. Vitamin C also increases interferon levels and functions as a potent antioxidant.

Although Dr. Pauling recommends dosages approaching 20,000 milligrams per day, most studies have shown significant antiviral benefit occurring at between 2,000 and 6,000 milligrams per day. It is also important to know that high doses of vitamin C can exacerbate or even precipitate loose bowel movements and diarrhea. As always, inform your primary care practitioner of any new therapies that you are utilizing. Even if there is not total agreement, he or she can advise you as to whether or not your individual condition might warrant extra caution.

Vitamin E

Vitamin E is primarily found in vegetable oils, leafy green vegetables, egg yolks, and whole grains. Its main function is to protect the body's cells from oxidation and free radical damage.

Simin Meydani, a nutritionist for the Department of Agriculture, recently presented the results of a study investigating the immune-stimulating effects of vitamin E. For her study, Meydani recruited thirty-four healthy volunteers and determined their level of immune response with standard skin tests and the measurement of white-blood-cell responses to foreign materials. Meydani then housed the thirty-four volunteers at the Department of Agriculture's Human Nutrition Resource Center in Boston for thirty days.

Group 1 was fed a normal diet containing 15 IU of vitamin E per day. Group 2 was fed the same diet plus daily supplementation with 800 IU of vitamin E. The study was set up so that neither the researchers nor the test subjects were aware of which group was receiving the additional vitamin E until the study results were reviewed.

After thirty days, the results of the study indicated that the group receiving the vitamin E supplementation had a *significant increase in their immune response* when compared to the unsupplemented group.

Additionally, studies at Tulane University suggest that vitamin E increases the anti-HIV activity of AZT. It accomplishes this by making cell membranes more permeable, thereby increasing the diffusion of AZT into infected cells. Accordingly, lower doses of AZT might be more effective when combined with this vitamin. It is also believed that Vitamin E may reduce the bone-marrow toxicity caused by AZT.

Vitamin E comes in several forms. The optimal forms of vitamin E supplementation are the natural, oil-based alpha-tocopherol or mixed tocopherol formulations (alpha, beta, gamma, and delta). These are the forms of vitamin E that have the highest biological activity and thus the most potential for enhancing the functioning of the immune system.

Beta Carotene/Vitamin A

Carotenoids make up more than 400 red and yellow pigments in nature. Beta carotene is the most plentiful in human foods. Beta carotene is also known as "provitamin A." It is converted to vitamin A in the gastrointestinal tract. The Recommended Dietary Allowance of vitamin A is 5,000 IU for adults and 2,500 IU for children. There is no specific RDA for beta carotene. This nutrient helps to maintain the integrity of the mucous membranes, fight infections, and detoxify air pollutants. It is required for the growth and repair of cells and is necessary for normal protein metabolism. It also serves as an antioxidant and helps protect the body against the growth of cancerous cells.

A deficiency of vitamin A can cause anemia, neurologic degeneration, dry skin, an inflamed tongue, gastrointestinal disorders, and the loss of taste and smell. The need for this nutrient is increased if you are under stress.

According to the most recent survey by the U.S. Department of Health, Education and Welfare, about 60 percent of women and 50 percent of men have intakes below the RDA for vitamin A. Although supplementing vitamin A in large doses can be toxic, the use of beta carotene supplements has never been shown to possess toxicity at any dosage level. When large doses of beta carotene are ingested, the only side effect is a yellowing of the skin pigment, which is not harmful and is reversible by decreasing the dose.

Beta carotene also demonstrates several positive effects not attributable to vitamin A. For instance, it has been shown to be more effective than vitamin A in the formation of healthy skin cells. It has also been shown to have an effect as an anticancer nutrient—a discovery made by the Japanese more than twenty years ago. Since then, many studies have validated the fact that people who eat an abundance of vegetables rich in beta carotene are less likely to develop cancers of the respiratory tract.

A study published in *Basic and Clinical Immunology* in 1982 showed that while modest increases in dietary vitamin A can enhance cell-mediated immunity, an excess of vitamin A depresses the immune response. This is a good reason to supplement your diet with beta carotene instead of vitamin A. When large doses of beta carotene are taken, the body utilizes only the amount it needs for vitamin A production. Since research has shown that beta carotene has its own immune-potentiating effects, it is the preferred method of supplementation for this nutrient.

Acidophilus Bacteria

One could call our intestinal bacteria "the elixir of good digestion." The intestinal tract of normal, healthy adults contains approximately 3½ pounds of bacteria. *Lactobacillus acidophilus* is a major component and helps to provide a beneficial environment for healthful digestion to occur. The equilibrium of beneficial intestinal bacteria may be disrupted by stress and by the use of many drugs. Since the majority of HIV-positive individuals will manifest some form of digestive imbalance at some time, daily acidophilus supplementation is suggested to help prevent these digestive problems from occurring.

Additional benefits of acidophilus supplementation include

- Production of significant amounts of B-complex vitamins, folic acid, and vitamin B_{12}.

- Reduction of intestinal gas and diarrhea.

- Improved digestion of dairy products due to an increased production of lactase.

If you are not yet convinced that there are significant benefits to be achieved by supplementing your diet with vitamins and other nutritional supplements, consider the following information:

- Numerous studies have linked vitamin and mineral deficiencies to weakened immune-system functioning. The most common deficiencies are of vitamins A, C, and E, zinc, and selenium.

- Many patients who have progressed to a diagnosis of AIDS have been shown to be deficient in both zinc and selenium.

- AZT use has been linked to low zinc levels in AIDS patients when compared to those not taking this drug.

- Malabsorption of vitamins and minerals from the digestive tract can be caused by antibiotic therapy, bacterial infections, intestinal parasites, and early HIV disease.

- Multiple studies have shown that dietary supplementation with vitamin A, vitamin C, vitamin E, beta carotene, and zinc enhances the cell-mediated arm of the immune system, which consists primarily of T-cells.

- T-helper cells have been shown to be stimulated by antioxidants such as beta carotene, vitamin C, vitamin E, zinc, selenium, and glutathione.

Since your immune system is the most sensitive system of your body to a nutrient deficiency, and since there is indisputable evidence that stress and the presence of a chronic infection raises the body's needs for many nutrients, doesn't it make sense to add vitamin and nutritional supplementation to your vitamin program?

Yes, it's hard work. But if you want to live and grow and remain healthy with HIV you must work a little harder than most to maintain your health. It has become your unique and special calling in life to learn how to stay healthy until a cure is found. You can do it! Get started today!

HERBS

Before the advent of our technologically based medical system, an abundance of natural substances were used to aid in the healing process. They included echinacea and goldenseal as antibiotics,

Figure 1.

(1989 Recommended Daily Allowances (RDA))

NUTRIENT	ADULT MALE	ADULT FEMALE
vitamin A	5,000 IU	5,000 IU
vitamin D	400 IU	400 IU
vitamin E	30 IU	30 IU
vitamin C	60 mg	60 mg
thiamine (B_1)	1.5 mg	1.1 mg
riboflavin (B_2)	1.7 mg	1.3 mg
niacin	19 mg	15 mg
folic acid	200 mcg	180 mcg
vitamin B_6	2 mg	1.6 mg
vitamin B_{12}	2 mcg	2 mcg
calcium	800 mg	800 mg (over age 50—1200 mg)
phosphorous	800 mg	800 mg
iron	10 mg	15 mg
zinc	15 mg	12 mg
magnesium	350 mg	280 mg
iodine	150 mcg	150 mcg
selenium	70 mcg	55 mcg
pantothenic acid	10 mg	10 mg
biotin	0.3 mg	0.3 mg

chamomile and valerian as sedatives, white willow bark and bayberry root for reducing fevers, and slippery elm and mint for curing indigestion and diarrhea.

Around the world, nature has provided an abundance of medicinal plants for healing. In fact, a 1975 survey showed that 74 percent of all prescription drugs worldwide were directly derived from plants. The main difference between natural substances and synthetic drugs is that synthetic drugs produce a quicker, stronger effect. Although the synthetic drugs may at times be lifesaving, they can also bring with them serious side effects. This is apparent when

Figure 2.

(Nutrients provided by four KAL Multi-Four tablets.)

VITAMINS

vitamin A (fish-liver oil)	10,000 IU
vitamin D (fish-liver oil)	400 IU
vitamin E (d-alpha-tocopherol)	200 IU
vitamin K (phytonadione)	50 mcg
vitamin C (calcium ascorbate)	500 mg
Bioflavonoids (citrus)	100 mg
Rutin	25 mg
Hesperidin	50 mg
folic acid	400 mcg
vitamin B_1 (thiamine HCl)	25 mg
vitamin B_2 (riboflavin)	25 mg
niacin	50 mg
niacinamide	100 mg
vitamin B_6 (pyridoxine HCl)	30 mg
vitamin B_{12} (cobalamin)	50 mcg
biotin	150 mcg
pantothenic acid	150 mg
(calcium d-pantothenate)	
choline (bitartrate)	200 mg
inositol	100 mg
para-aminobenzoic acid	30 mg

MINERALS

calcium (amino acid chelate)	500 mg
iodine (from kelp)	225 mcg
iron (amino acid chelate)	20 mg
magnesium (amino acid chelate)	250 mg
copper (amino acid chelate)	2 mg
zinc (amino acid chelate)	25 mg
manganese (amino acid chelate)	25 mg
potassium (amino acid proteinate)	50 mg

chromium (amino acid chelate)	50 mcg
selenium (L-selenomethionine)	25 mcg
DIGESTIVE AIDS	
iron ox bile	25 mg
bromelain	25 mg
pancrelipase	30 mg
papain	25 mg
betaine HCl	25 mg
HERBS	
alfalfa herb	65 mg
almond powder	65 mg
bladder wrack	65 mg
cascara sagrada	65 mg
cayenne	65 mg
comfrey herb	75 mg
dandelion root	65 mg
goldenseal root	65 mg
horsetail grass	65 mg
saw palmetto berries	65 mg
yellow dock	65 mg
MISCELLANEOUS	
RNA	50 mg
desiccated liver concentrate (defatted)	100 mg
lecithin	150 mg

one considers that the amount of medication necessary to adequately treat HIV is often toxic to its host. This dilemma is disturbing to anyone interested in a *nontoxic* approach to HIV treatment.

The Comprehensive Healing Program for HIV is designed to support the body's own ability to keep HIV dormant. The suggested herbs can help nurture and strengthen your body and immune system. Medications are utilized only when necessary and

Figure 3.

(Vitamins and nutritional supplements with potential side effects.)

NUTRIENT	DOSAGE	POTENTIAL SIDE EFFECT
vitamin A	greater than 100,000 IU/day	nausea, vomiting, liver damage
vitamin C	greater than 10 g/day	diarrhea
vitamin E	greater than 1,200 IU/day	high blood pressure, headaches
vitamin B_6	greater than 300 mg/day	peripheral neuropathy
zinc	greater than 100 mg/day	immune-system depression
selenium	greater than 200 mcg/day	immune-system depression

in dosages that provide beneficial effects without adverse side effects.

I have found that many of my patients who follow the herbal recommendations of this program require much lower dosages of medications such as AZT, ddI, and ddC, while continuing to remain stable and in good health. In fact, it is rare for my patients to take more than 300 mg of AZT per day while achieving the same results, if not better, than what is usually achieved with 500 mg or more. I believe this is due to the fact that the immune system is being supported and strengthened in many other ways. The body therefore requires less medication to achieve a beneficial effect without adverse side effects. Patients following the herbal recommendations of the Comprehensive Healing Program for HIV report fewer symptoms, a greater energy level, and an enhanced sense of well-being. The majority of them remain healthy and asymptomatic for extremely long periods of time.

In this section, I will present information that describes herbs from both the Western and Oriental schools of thought. Herbs can be utilized in two ways. First, they can be used as tonics, that is, to enhance the functioning of the immune system, promote beneficial circulation, restore energy, and normalize physiologic processes. Second, herbs can be used as initial remedies for minor symptoms. In the Comprehensive Healing Program for HIV, traditional Oriental herbs provide the core of the program, while Western herbs are used in a supplemental fashion. *Under no circumstances should herbal remedies be used as the sole treatment for the HIV infection.* An intelligent blend of both natural and standard medical therapies provides the optimal approach for treating HIV.

I recommend that you choose a few herbs from the following list that address your particular concerns (i.e. immune system strengthening, digestive aid, sleep aid, etc.). These should then be added to the traditional Oriental herbal formula described later in this chapter.

The following three books may prove valuable to anyone interested in a more expanded and detailed discussion of herbal medicine:

1. *The Scientific Validation of Herbal Medicine,* by Daniel B. Mowrey, Ph.D., Cormorant Books 1986

2. *The Way of Herbs,* by Michael Tierra C.A., N.D., Washington Square Press 1983

3. *The Male Herbal,* by James Green, The Crossing Press 1991

Western Antibiotic Herbs

Western herbs that contain antibiotic and antiviral properties have been used for centuries by herbalists in the successful treatment of many types of bacterial and viral infections. These herb possess many nutrients as well as antibiotic and antiviral components. They are excellent for general use as tonics or, in higher dosages, for the treatment of acute infections.

Echinacea

Echinacea angustifolia has been used in the Americas and Western Europe for hundreds of years to strengthen the immune system. Its major component, inulin, helps promote the movement of white blood cells toward an infection (chemotaxis). It also promotes the solubilization of antibody-virus complexes that need to be cleansed from the bloodstream. Echinacea also possesses a direct antiviral effect. Mammalian cells treated with extracts of echinacea have been shown to be 50 to 80 percent resistant to influenza, herpes, and oral stomatitis viruses.

Recent pharmacological investigations support the fact that echinacea is an immune-stimulating agent. A substance known as echinacin has been shown to be a T-cell and macrophage stimulator. It stimulates the production of interferon as well as other lymphokines.

Echinacea is probably the best detoxifying agent of any herb known to Western herbalists. Michael Tierra, author of *The Way of Herbs,* calls it "the most effective blood and lymphatic cleanser in the botanical kingdom." It is gentle and does not have any side effects.

Recommended dosage: 25 to 40 drops of high-quality organic echinacea tincture *or* 2 to 3 capsules of the dried herb, three times a day. For acute ailments this dose is best taken every one to two hours for maximum benefit. Side effects: none.

Goldenseal Root

Goldenseal root is frequently used to help reduce inflammation and treat infections. It has been found to be effective for use as a restorative herb following protracted fevers. The alkaloids present in this herb, especially berberine and hydrastine, have been used to combat a wide variety of infections.

A study done in India showed that berberine has a protective effect against intestinal amoebic infections in rats. Other Indian studies demonstrated a similar but even more pronounced effect against cholera bacteria. Goldenseal extract has been shown to be effective against gram-positive bacteria, such as staph and strep, and against gram-negative bacteria, such as *E. coli.* Additionally, the alkaloids in goldenseal root show the ability to inhibit the growth of tuberculosis organisms. Goldenseal has been found to cure intestinal parasitic infections such as giardiasis, which has been a major problem in Africa and Asia and is beginning to surface more and more frequently in Western countries, including the United States.

Goldenseal root is a powerful herb, and it should not be taken in large amounts or for prolonged periods of time. Two or three capsules a day of the dried root powder is generally considered safe and adequate for most conditions. Excessive use of goldenseal can diminish B-vitamin absorption because of its antibiotic effect against favorable intestinal bacteria. Therefore, you should supplement your diet with acidophilus bacteria if you are taking goldenseal root.

Recommended dosage: 2 to 3 capsules or 1 to 2 dropperfuls of organic tincture once per day. Zand's Echinacea/Goldenseal formula (Insure Herbal) and Rainbow Light's Vitamune tincture provide beneficial combination formulas that contain Goldenseal root. These herbal tinctures, taken in moderation, can be effectively used as a general immune system tonic. You may increase the dosage for up to one week if any acute symptoms such as fevers, night sweats, or excessive mucus production are present. Side effects: nausea, rash, and inhibition of intestinal bacterial growth.

Myrrh

Myrrh is a potent herbal antiseptic. It is often combined with Goldenseal to make an antibiotic salve. A tincture of myrrh makes an excellent mouthwash for painful, bleeding gums. Myrrh is commonly used as an external treatment because it contains volatile oils that are toxic when taken in large amounts internally; however, it possesses detoxifying qualities and can be taken internally in small amounts to treat indigestion and excessive intestinal gas. It is also an excellent treatment for chronic catarrh (mucus production) and bronchial congestion. I would recommend taking an acidophilus supplement if you are taking myrrh internally.

Recommended dosage: 1 to 2 capsules or 30 drops of high-quality tincture up to three times a day, not to exceed a duration of one week for the treatment of acute conditions. The tincture can also be mixed with water and used as a mouthwash. The salve may be used up to four times a day externally. Do not apply the salve to mucous membranes or near your eyes. Side effects: nausea and inhibition of intestinal bacterial growth.

Garlic

The list of medicinal effects attributed to garlic is long and well documented. Garlic helps lower cholesterol levels, decreases high blood pressure, helps to prevent strokes, and inhibits the growth of many pathogenic microorganisms including bacteria, fungi, and viruses.

The active ingredient in fresh garlic is called allicin. It is the key antibacterial and antiviral agent. It is also the chemical that gives garlic its notorious odor. Because onions, botanical cousins to garlic, also contain allicin, they possess similar properties. Dr. Byron Murray, head of the virus research laboratory at Brigham Young University in Utah, states that garlic, in high concentrations, kills viruses more effectively than alcohol, acetone, and most common disinfectants.

Garlic's antibacterial activity has been proven against numerous bacteria including staph, strep, *Klebsiella, Proteus, E. coli, Salmonella* and *Vibrio cholera.* Of major significance are the antifungal studies that show garlic to be effective against *Candida albicans,* the organism responsible for thrush, and *Tinea,* the organism which causes athlete's foot and ringworm. At least twenty other pathogenic fungi are susceptible to either inhibition or destruction by garlic.

Additionally, garlic is extremely nutritious and contains high levels of protein, vitamin A, vitamin C, thiamine, and many minerals including copper, zinc, iron, calcium, potassium, sulfur, and selenium.

In 1980, a study was performed in China with eleven patients who had contracted cryptococcal meningitis. The patients were treated with garlic extract orally and by injection, either intramuscularly or intravenously, over a period of several weeks. Side effects were minimal and all eleven patients recovered successfully. This study was reported in the *Chinese Medical Journal* and was entitled "Garlic and Cryptococcal Meningitis: A Preliminary Report." Although this study shows that garlic has powerful antifungal effects, I would strongly suggest using it more for preventive therapy than as treatment for acute conditions.

Recommended dosage: An abundance of fresh garlic and onions should be included in the diet. If desired, supplement your diet with 2 to 8 garlic capsules per day. In my experience, Nature's Way Garlicin has had extensive scientific investigation by an independent laboratory and is highly potent. Side effects: indigestion, halitosis.

Digestive Aids

Chamomile

Chamomile is known in Europe as a "cure-all." Leading the list of its proven properties is an antispasmodic effect helpful in reducing irritable bowel symptoms. One of the best established properties of chamomile is its antiinflammatory effect. It can be applied internally or externally to decrease inflammation. It can also be used on the gums to relieve swelling and pain.

Chamomile beneficially affects the nerves, stomach, kidneys, and liver. It is known as a diaphoretic (it encourages sweating to help break fevers) and a potent sedative. It has antibacterial and antifungal effects and is also useful for treating dermatologic ailments. It has a mild stimulating effect on the liver.

Recommended dosage: A medicinal tea can be made by steeping one-quarter ounce of chamomile in a pint of boiled water for ten minutes. Chamomile tincture can also be used 1 to 2 tablespoons at a time, one to three times daily. Externally, chamomile can be applied to swellings, sore muscles, and painful joints as a poultice— a warm, moistened pack of herbs that is held to the skin by a clean cotton bandage. Side effects: none.

Slippery Elm

Slippery-elm bark can be used internally and externally for soothing mucous membranes. This herb is extremely effective for sore throats, bronchitis, and sinusitis when used as a tea. It is also very soothing to the digestive system.

Slippery elm was originally used by the American Indians and Western settlers to treat urinary and bowel irritation, scurvy, dysentery, and ulcers. It was applied externally as a poultice for tumors, burns, and open wounds. The active ingredient in slippery-elm bark is mucilage, which is the soluble fiber responsible for the herb's soothing action. In the treatment of HIV, slippery elm can be used to treat coughs, bronchitis, and any malabsorptive conditions of the digestive tract.

Recommended dosage: Slippery elm is best used internally in combination with other herbs. A traditional formula for treating colitis is ½ teaspoon of slippery elm bark powder added to 1 cup of chamomile or peppermint tea, sweetened to taste with honey. Drink the tea slowly and repeat several times a day. Side effects: diarrhea and bloating *if taken in excessive amounts.*

Peppermint, Spearmint, and Catnip

Peppermint is probably the best known of the mints. Its use can be traced back to the beginnings of recorded history. Its essential oils enhance digestive action by stimulating the gallbladder to secrete bile. It has been shown to reduce intestinal gas and alleviate cramping. Recent research has attributed antiulcer and antiinflammatory properties to peppermint. Peppermint has also been shown to inhibit and kill many kinds of bacteria and viruses that can cause digestive imbalances. Studies have been published showing peppermint's inhibitory effect on the following organisms: influenza A virus, herpes simplex virus, mumps virus; strep, staph, and *Pseudomonas* bacteria; and *Candida albicans* yeast.

Peppermint is the most mentally stimulating of the mints and the best for improving digestion. Spearmint is more relaxing and has a diuretic action. Catnip, often called catmint, has many of the same properties as peppermint. It is soothing to the gastrointestinal tract and is often used to treat infant colic. Like peppermint, it has been shown to have antibiotic properties, although its research is not nearly as extensive. Catnip is sometimes called "nature's Alka-Seltzer," although this term is applicable to all of the mints.

Recommended dosage: ¼ ounce of herb, steeped in 1 pint of boiled water for 10 minutes. This produces an infusion (steeped tea) with the above-mentioned medicinal benefits. Side effects: none.

Nervines

Nervines are herbs that strengthen and relax the nervous system. Since stress reduction is important for a healthy immune system, these herbs can be a beneficial part of your program.

The nervine family includes chamomile, hops, valerian, skullcap, and passion flower. These herbs work best when used in combination. They are taken as teas, capsules, or tinctures. Find the product that helps you relax the best. Use it to balance and strengthen your nervous system so that you can cultivate the inner calm necessary for good health and healing. Side effects: none.

Oriental Herbs

Chinese Tonic Herbs

Chinese tonic herbs have been used for centuries to protect the body from external diseases. In addition to keeping the immune system strong, Chinese tonic herbs help tone and balance the *chi,* or energy flow of the body.

These herbs have very potent effects when taken individually. However, the major benefit of most herbal preparations stems from their use in effective combinations. These combinations bring together herbs from different categories into effective, balanced formulas. A combination of different herbs usually addresses the needs of the body more effectively than a single remedy.

Listed below are general descriptions of the seven most important Chinese tonic herbs found in RESIST, a product which has been studied as part of the Comprehensive Healing Program for HIV Research Study since 1988. The ingredients in RESIST are based upon a thoroughly tested Chinese tonic formula that has been slightly modified based on current research findings. RESIST is distributed by Pacific BioLogic, a company based in Orinda, California, which has proven, during the past five years, to be committed to bringing the highest-quality Chinese herbs to its customers and has supported the Comprehensive Healing Program for HIV since its inception. As you will see, there has been extensive animal and human testing done with all of the herbs listed. Much of it substantiates that they are powerful natural substances possessing many immune-strengthening properties.

Unfortunately, the research conducted in China and other foreign countries is often not completely accepted by American researchers. This is partially due to the fact that the Chinese medical system utilizes concepts and descriptive terms unfamiliar to most Western researchers (*chi,* meridians, energy flow, cooling and heating effects, and so on). I hope that as both the Oriental and Western schools of medical thought share their findings, a truly universal system of medical treatment more effective than either alone will begin to emerge. This philosophy is already being implemented in China, where Western drugs *and* herbal treatments are combined in the treatment of diseases such as cancer, heart disease, and diabetes with excellent results.

The following description of Chinese tonic herbs and their properties was taken with permission from the work of Subhuti Dharmananda, Ph.D., the director of the Institute for Traditional Medicine and Preventive Health Care in Portland, Oregon. Much of it is from a paper he wrote entitled "Chinese Herbal Therapies for the Treatment of Immunodeficiency Syndromes," printed in the January 1987 issue of the *Oriental Healing Arts International Bulletin.* Dr. Dharmananda has been a pioneer for many years in the field of traditional Chinese herbal therapy and specializes in the treatment of HIV and other immunodeficiency syndromes. A list of practitioners who specialize in using Chinese herbs for the adjunctive treatment of immunodeficiency states is available by writing to the Institute for Traditional Medicine (ITM), 2017 SE Hawthorne, Portland, OR 97214.

Astragalus

Astragalus is the dried root of *Astragalus membranaceus,* a perennial attaining a height of about 20 feet and grown in northern China. This herb is now being cultivated commercially. After the roots are dug up, the outsides are briefly fired to remove the small rootlets, and the material is sliced diagonally to produce long, thin slats. The yellow color of the interior is used as a measure of the quality of the herb.

The following components are responsible for astragalus's active effects: polysaccharides, gluconic acid, mucilage, amino acids, choline, betaine, folic acid, kumatakenin, and flavones, including quercetin, isorhamnepin, and ramnocitrin.

Several specific fractions of polysaccharides are believed to be responsible for its major immune-stimulating effects. These fractions, when injected into rats, increase the number of macrophages, enhance T-cell transformation (from suppressors to helpers), and increase phagocytosis. In mice, astragalus promotes the ability of the immune system to produce interferon and increases the clearing rate of toxins.

Human clinical trials have demonstrated that when astragalus is given to cancer patients receiving chemotherapy or radiation therapy, a substantial increase in one-, three-, and five-year survival rates is observed. Astragalus has also been shown to increase the number of antibodies (IgA and IgG) in the blood and to induce the production of interferon by white blood cells.

According to traditional Chinese medicine, astragalus is classified as a warm, sweet tonic that enhances the functioning of the spleen and lung. It is recommended for general strengthening, treating excessive perspiration, eliminating toxins, and promoting the healing of damaged tissues. It is commonly used for the treatment of edema, night sweats, skin ulcerations, and abscesses. Pure astragalus root is sometimes processed by cooking with honey in order to enhance its effect and palatability. The cooked astragalus can be used for the treatment of lethargy, weak digestion, anemia, and poor appetite. Astragalus can also be taken as a decoction (the liquid fraction after boiling the root in water for half an hour) or combined with other herbs in powder form as pills, tablets, or capsules. The typical dosage of this combination formula is about 9 grams per day, of which astragalus traditionally comprises 15 to 20 percent of the total.

Schizandra

Schizandra is the ripe fruit of *Schizandra sinensis.* This plant is a woody vine that is generally found climbing treetops by twining around the trunks. It is native to the mountain forests of northern China, and commercial cultivation is currently only at the experimental stage. During the fall, the ripe fruit is collected and sun dried to prevent mildew. Schizandra is a stimulant herb, found to affect the central nervous system of both animals and human beings. Clinical evaluations have shown that it enhances energy level and mental acuity. It is thus helpful in overcoming stress and fatigue and in enhancing one's performance at work.

Several studies involving schizandra were reported at an international conference in Hong Kong in 1984. Schizandra extract was proven successful for the treatment of a number of hepatitis syndromes, including viral hepatitis. In animals, its effects include protection of liver cells from fatty degeneration and an enhancement of lymphocyte transformation. In patients with chronic hepatitis, schizandra has been proven to lower the production of liver enzymes (AST, ALT) in about 80 percent of the cases as well as producing overall improvement in a majority of clinical symptoms.

In traditional Chinese medicine, Schizandra is regarded as a warm, astringent tonic. It is classically used as a Chi tonic for the Lungs and Kidneys to treat edema, sweating, and chronic diarrhea. Schizandra is frequently combined with other herbs that nurture the Yin and Essence and used in the treatment of exhaustion, weight loss, and thirst. The dosage for Shizandra ranges from 3 to 20 grams per day depending on the condition to be treated.

Ligustrum

Ligustrum is derived from the fruit of the *Ligustrum lucidium* plant, which is found throughout many parts of the Far East. In China, ligustrum is mostly collected throughout the Sichuan province. The plant is an evergreen shrub that grows to about thirteen feet in height, producing clusters of black berries. The fruit contains the following active ingredients: syringin, oleanolic acid, demanite, osolic acid, nueshenide, and oleuropenin.

Ligustrum has been used for several centuries in China as a tonic for the kidneys. Like astragalus, this herb is used as a tonic when there has been a rapid deterioration of the body, such as occurs when the immune system is failing.

Ligustrum is a diuretic and a cardiac stimulant. It inhibits the growth of bacteria and has been shown to raise the white-blood-cell count of patients undergoing cancer therapies. As a measure of its ability to stimulate the immune system, mononuclear cells from thirteen cancer patients were treated with ligustrum extract. The graft-versus-host reaction, a measure of the immune system's reactivity, converted from negative to positive in nine of the thirteen patients.

In traditional Chinese medicine, ligustrum is classified as a yin tonic. It is used in the treatment of aging, dizziness, tinnitus, backache, and blurred vision. It has a sweet, bitter taste with cooling properties. It is usually prepared as a decoction, about 6 to 15 grams per day. Alcohol extracts and tablets of this herb have also been used in clinical practice with success.

Ganoderma

Ganoderma is a fungus of the *Ganoderma lucidium* family. This family yields many important Chinese herbs and is also famous in Japan, where it is known as the reishi mushroom. The fungus grows on old, broadleaf trees and often attains a weight of over a pound. Ganoderma is relatively rare and thus costly, but commercial cultivation has brought the price down considerably. The most useful form of the mushroom is the rare antler form, which has many branches and spores rather than a single cap. Recently a technique for growing ganoderma with a high spore content has been developed in Japan.

Ganoderma contains polysaccharides that are known to enhance the functioning of the immune system. In laboratory studies, these polysaccharides suppress the growth of implanted tumor cells. The mechanism of action involves an increase in T-cell and macrophage activity.

In the treatment of viral hepatitis, ganoderma has been shown to improve symptoms such as anorexia, insomnia, malaise, and liver swelling. In one study, the AST liver enzymes decreased in 70 percent of the patients.

Ganoderma is a stress-reducing herb effective in treating conditions such as stomach ulcers and high blood pressure. In persons suffering insomnia, it enhances the relaxation of muscles and increases sleeping time. It also reduces lipids and cholesterol in the blood.

Traditionally, ganoderma has been used in China as a *chi* tonic and sedative. The taste is sweet and slightly bitter. It is usually taken in doses of 9 to 15 grams prepared as a decoction, although doses as low as 4 to 6 grams daily have proven effective for the treatment of insomnia, nervousness, and chronic infections. It can be made into pills in combination with other herbs and represents 10 to 20 percent of the mixture. Liquid extracts of ganoderma have recently been manufactured in China and are often mixed with other *chi* tonics.

White Atractylodes

White atractylodes is the dried root of *Atractylodes macrocephala*. It is a perennial herb, growing one to three feet in height. It is generally found growing in the Zhejian, Jiangxi, Hunan, Hubei, and Shanxi provinces of China. The wild plant is scarce; the herb found on the market is derived from commercial cultivation. It is grown in sandy soil that is well drained and fertilized with organic material. White atractylodes is differentiated from "ordinary atractylodes," a less expensive herb from another member of the *Atractylodes* family.

Important constituents of white atractylodes are elemol, atractylol, and atractylon, which are found in the volatile oils. The herb also contains vitamin A and has been proven useful in treating night blindness caused by vitamin A deficiency.

As an immune-stimulating agent, white atractylodes has been shown to be beneficial in enhancing the phagocytic functions of white blood cells and to help increase their numbers. It is an important component in several classic immune-enhancing formulas and is usually combined with astragalus and/or ginseng for maximum effect.

White atractylodes is a diuretic. In one study, a dose of 0.05 to 0.25 grams per kilogram of body weight of the decoction liquid injected intravenously into dogs resulted in excretion of urine nearly nine times the level of controls during a five-hour period.

Laboratory experiments have demonstrated the tonic effect of white atractylodes. In oral administration of the decoction for one month, laboratory animals showed increases in body weight and enhanced physical endurance. It has also been shown to have a protective effect on the liver against damage by chemical toxins.

According to traditional Chinese medicine, white atractylodes is a sweet and bitter warming tonic for the spleen and stomach. It is used to rid the body of excessive moisture, improve digestion, increase apetite, and lessen fatigue. It has also been used as therapy for dizziness, diarrhea, and night sweats. The dosage used to make a decoction is 5 to 10 grams. The herb is also made into pills in combination with other herbs and commonly comprises 10 to 40 percent of the mixture.

Codonopsis

Codonopsis is the root of the *Codonopsis pilosula* plant, which grows in northern China and is cultivated in the Sichuan and Hubei provinces. The perennial herb grows to approximately three feet in height. The roots, collected in the fall, are graded by size. The active constituents of this herb are saponins and alkaloids.

Codonopsis is used throughout China as a substitute for the more expensive ginseng. It is considered to have nearly identical properties to ginseng but to have less effect of "heating the blood."

It is therefore the preferred herb for use in the treatment of HIV disease, a condition known for its excess dampness and heat. Codonopsis is also considered to have a somewhat greater effect than ginseng on the lungs. It is in the same family as three other lung-active herbs: platycodon, adenophora, and lobelia. While ginseng has been amply tested and proven effective as an immune enhancer in both Korea and the Soviet Union, codonopsis has been evaluated only more recently. Like ginseng, it has shown to be beneficial in the treatment of laboratory animals and human patients undergoing cancer therapies.

Codonopsis stimulates the growth of red blood cells, enhances T-cell transformation, and stimulates phagocytosis. The combination of ganoderma, astragalus and codonopsis has been shown to enhance phagocytosis and promote lymphocyte transformation. In a study of its immune-stimulating effects, codonopsis was used as the main ingredient in combination with white atractylodes and hoelen. This mixture enhanced the rate of rosette formation of lymphocytes in the blood, a measure of their stimulation. It also increased the level of IgG antibodies in the bloodstream.

In traditional Chinese medicine, codonopsis is classified as a neutral-energy, sweet *chi* tonic used for disorders of the spleen and lungs. It has been used in the treatment of heart palpitations, nervousness, menstrual disorders, and breast cancer. The usual dose is 9 to 15 grams taken as a decoction. It can also be used in pills, representing 10 to 25 percent of the mixture.

Licorice

Licorice is one of the most widely used herbs in Chinese medicine. It is derived from the root and lower stem of *Glycyrrhiza uralensis* and *Glycyrrhiza glabra*. Much of the Chinese licorice supply is from northern China, especially from Heilong Jiang Province.

The plant is a shrub that grows to a height of two to three feet. The dried root slices are frequently processed with honey to enhance the herb's *chi*-strengthening effect.

The principle active constituents of licorice are saponin glycosides. The sweet taste of licorice is due to glycyrrhizin, which is rated fifty times sweeter per unit weight than sugar. Glycyrrhizin has been shown to be effective in treating acute and chronic viral hepatitis. In one study, 85 percent of the patients receiving it experienced clinical cure and the remainder showed marked improvement. In contrast, only 35 percent of the twenty-person control group, receiving a different therapy, were cured. In addition, glycyrrhizin has been shown to produce increases in IgG, IgA and IgM antibody levels.

Licorice root's effects with regard to the treatment of fevers and infections has been clearly substantiated. One study in China found that licorice root possessed antibacterial activity against several common gram-negative intestinal bacteria. Later, in 1979, a team of Italian researchers reported a series of experiments in which they discovered several antiviral effects attributable to licorice root. These included the extracellular destruction of virus particles, the prevention of intracellular virus activation, and the impairment of the assembly of viral components. Recent experiments in China have revealed that licorice root activates the body's interferon mechanism. In the United States, a team of investigators has recently reported study results verifying licorice root's antimicrobial properties against *Staphyloccus* and *Mycobacterium* species. *Mycobacterium* species are responsible for MAI and tuberculosis infections and are now the second leading cause of opportunistic infections in AIDS patients.

Licorice root is an important component of many Chinese herbal combinations and is classified as a sweet, neutral-energy *chi* tonic. It may be used as a decoction, in doses of up to 24 grams for the treatment of laryngitis, coughing spasms, and severe pain. It usually comprises about 5 percent of general tonic formulas and works to potentiate other herbs in the combination.

The RESIST Formula

Traditional Chinese herbalists prepare decoctions (the tea made from boiling herbs in water for half an hour) using as much as 20 to 30 grams of dried herb per day. In order to reduce the amount of the tea that must be consumed, the makers of RESIST employ a sophisticated concentration method to reduce the hot water preparation into highly concentrated granules which are then encapsulated. Since RESIST is a 4 to 1 concentrate, each 750-milligram capsule provides similar potency to 3 grams of dried herbs. The dosage of RESIST in the Comprehensive Healing Program is 12 capsules per day. This is equivalent to 36 grams of dried herb per day. This dosage may be modified based on an individual's needs once therapy has begun. If you have any questions regarding the use of Chinese herbs as part of your healing program, it is recommended that you consult a physician or acupuncturist trained in the practice of Oriental medicine before embarking upon therapy.

RESIST Dosage: 4 capsules taken three times a day on an empty stomach with water or other fluid.

RESIST Formula

EACH CONCENTRATED 750-MILLIGRAM CAPSULE CONTAINS THE EQUIVALENT OF THE FOLLOWING AMOUNTS OF CRUDE HERBS:

Astragalus	390 mg
Ganoderma mushroom	240 mg
Codonopsis root	285 mg
Atractylodes	180 mg
Licorice root	135 mg
Rehmannia	180 mg
Sand root	180 mg
Schizandra	143 mg
Ginger root	143 mg
Jujube fruit	143 mg
Millettia root	180 mg
Dodder seeds	180 mg
Chinese yam root	180 mg
Balloon flower root	143 mg
Ligustrum	180 mg
Peony root	90 mg
Tangerine peel	90 mg

Side effects: RESIST has very few side effects. The formula possesses an overall warming quality so care should be taken if an inflammatory condition, such as chronic sinusitis, colitis, or dermatitis, is present. If you have any doubts, work up to the recommended dosage slowly (over two to three weeks) while closely observing for any adverse effects. It is also recommended that occasional breaks be taken from herbal tonic formulas such as RESIST to prevent the body from becoming tolerant to its effects. My recommendation is one month off to every three months on. Zand's Insure Herbal formula, containing echinacea and goldenseal, can be substituted for RESIST at a dosage of 3 tablets twice a day during this one-month break. Once again, consider consulting a trained health professional for guidance if you have any specific questions regarding your herbal regimen. RESIST may be obtained from Pacific BioLogic Inc. 108 Camino Pablo Road, Orinda, CA 94563 (800) 869-8783.

Fu Zheng Therapy

The RESIST formula is based on a traditional Chinese form of healing known as *fu zheng* therapy. Literally this means "to restore normalcy and balance to the body."

In practice, *fu zheng* therapy does not specifically treat an infective agent but works toward rebuilding the resistance of the individual. Its goal is to enable the body to rebuild its strength and balance so as to more effectively contend with both the causes of a disease and the manifestations of that disease.

Initial interest by Western medical researchers in *fu zheng* therapy can be traced back to research papers published by investigators at the Department of Medical Oncology at Beijing Cancer Institute in 1982. Clinicians there reported significant increases in the survival rates of cancer patients receiving a combination of *fu zheng* herbs and conventional therapies, such as radiation and chemotherapy. There was a notable decrease in the immunosuppressive effects of these therapies when *fu zheng* herbs were added to the standard medical regimen. Following the evaluation of several *fu zheng* combinations, two principal herbs were chosen for use as adjuncts to conventional therapies at the Beijing Cancer Institute. These were astragalus and ligustrum, two of the principle herbs used in the RESIST formula.

ADDITIONAL STUDIES IN HIV-POSITIVE PATIENTS

There have been several other studies utilizing *fu zheng* herbs for the treatment of the HIV condition. One of these studies was performed by U.S. herbalist Subhuti Dharmananda in 1986. He and two other herbalists, Susan Black and Jay Sordean, developed a protocol for determining whether Chinese herbs might be helpful for persons with ARC or AIDS.

The Immune Enhancement Project treated twenty ARC patients for a period exceeding three months. Most of the participants were symptomatic and therefore able to report whether *fu zheng* therapy was helpful in diminishing their symptoms. The basic herbal combinations used in the Immune Enhancement Project consisted of an astragalus-based formula, known as Astra 8, designed by Dr. Dharmananda, and a second formula prepared from *shiitaki* and cascade mushrooms from Portland, Oregon. Once a month, participants filled out a questionnaire consisting of a lengthy checklist of symptoms. There was improvement in all twenty of the patients. Diarrhea and night sweats were virtually eliminated, and energy levels were improved in all but two of the participants. There was no control group.

A second study utilizing *fu zheng* therapy was conducted by the Quan Yin Center for Healing Arts in San Francisco. This study, originally designed by herbalist Misha Cohen, also showed a decrease in symptoms and an overall improvement in most patients' energy levels. Some very ill patients were even able to return to work after adding Chinese herbs to their program of standard medical therapies.

Most recently, studies performed at the University of Texas System Cancer Center, M. D. Anderson Hospital and Tumor Institute, by Drs. Chu, Wong, Mavligit, and others, have shown that purified fractions of astragalus root possess potent immune-restorative activity both in the test tube and in rats. Dr. Chu and his coworkers have found that by incubating astragalus extract and white blood cells along with interleukin-2, a naturally produced immune mediator, they produced a tenfold increase in the white blood cells' ability to kill tumor cells. Since interleukin-2 is toxic when given to patients in high doses, the researchers hope that simultaneous use of astragalus purified fractions and interleukin-2 will allow smaller, less toxic dosages of interleukin-2 to be used while yielding superior results.

In another paper from M. D. Anderson Hospital and Tumor Institute, Dr. Chu concluded that

> *a failing immune system in human subjects, manifested by deficient T-cell function from debilitating diseases such as cancer or AIDS, may be partially restored or augmented to a certain extent by various biological response modifiers. . . . Our data distinctly indicates that either the crude extract of* Astragalus membranaceus, *or its column separated fraction #3, can completely restore a failing immune system and bring its T-cell's functioning, in vitro, to the normal level found among cells derived from healthy subjects. The properties possessed by this traditional Chinese medicinal herbal extract renders it an important biological response modifier which should be considered for clinical trials of immunotherapy in persons who suffer from primary or secondary immunologic deficiency and its associated serious complications.*

Many of Dr. Chu's papers, including the above passage, were published in the *Journal of Clinical Laboratory Immunology* in 1988. As you probably know, there has not been a mad dash to begin studying the effects of astragalus and its purified fractions in AIDS patients, even as an adjunct to AZT. In fact, there are only a few studies throughout the United States that are in the process of testing Chinese herbs as an adjunct to the standard treatment of HIV. One of these studies is being conducted at San Francisco

General Hospital. Its purpose is to find out if Chinese medicinal herbs can help reduce the symptoms and improve the overall well-being of people with HIV. It will compare Chinese herbs to a placebo in HIV-positive individuals with between 200 and 500 T-helper cells during a twelve-week period. At the end of the study, patients who were taking the placebo will be given a free twelve-week supply of the Chinese herbs, if they wish to take them. Interested individuals may contact the SFGH AIDS Research Group at (415) 476-9296, ext. 84602 to find out if this study is still open to enrollment at the time of this publication.

Hopefully, as additional data surfaces to highlight the benefits that herbs can bring to HIV care, more research funding will be channeled in the direction of investigating these potent and beneficial medicines.

Summary

I have discussed many useful herbs in this chapter. The most common regimen that I prescribe for my HIV positive patients is as follows:

1. RESIST: 4 capsules three times a day for three months, followed by a one-month break. Zand's Insure Herbal formula, at a dosage of 3 tablets, two times a day, may be substituted for RESIST during this break. Then, begin this rotation again.

2. Western antibiotic herbs (echinacea, goldenseal, garlic and others) may be taken on a rotating basis for their general toning effects.

3. Additional Western and Oriental herbs as needed for the specific treatment of minor ailments (as prescribed by your health-care practitioner).

It is important to realize that these herbs should comprise *one component* of an overall treatment program that includes a healthful diet, vitamins, exercise, stress reduction, and, when indicated, standard medications. This type of overall approach will enable your herbal program to work much more effectively. The Comprehensive Healing Program for HIV should be viewed as a combination approach. The immune strengthening value of each of the individual therapies potentiates the other therapies. This enables the overall program to more effectively keep HIV dormant.

EXERCISE

Check the box that applies to you:

☐ I make no effort to obtain regular exercise.

☐ I live an active life and get my workouts from daily living activities such as walking, climbing stairs, shopping, and running for the bus.

☐ I make a modest effort to obtain regular exercise (one to three times weekly).

☐ I obtain regular exercise three to five times per week (at least thirty minutes per session).

☐ I obtain regular exercise greater than five times per week (at least thirty minutes per sesson).

If you checked the box stating that you live an active life but do not get any regular exercise, you are not providing your body with the stimulation that it needs for the optimal functioning of your immune system. Regular exercise is necessary to *enhance* the functioning of the immune system. The Comprehensive Healing Program for HIV recommends that an asymptomatic HIV-positive individual exercise three to five times per week for at least thirty minutes per session. Symptomatic individuals should not exert themselves more than feels comfortable.

It is extremely important that you *enjoy* the exercise activities that you practice. If you enjoy them, you will look forward to them. Enjoyable exercise can become a wonderful outlet for stress, a source of personal satisfaction, and an invigorating physical release.

When you are deciding which exercises to make part of your Comprehensive Healing Program, remember that it is important to achieve the following goals:

1. *Deep breathing:* During exercise, deep breathing helps cleanse the lungs. It also acts as a pump for the lymphatic system. Lymph is a milky fluid made up of water, protein, antibodies, and white blood cells. It flows through the lymphatic channels, which parallel the circulatory system. It passes through the lymph nodes and cleanses them. *It is the lifeblood of your immune system.*

Your lymph nodes become swollen because they are congested with material that has been cleansed from your tissues and bloodstream, including dead cells, bacteria, and virus particles. To help relieve this congestion, lymph is pushed through the system by deep breathing and the pumping action of your muscles.

Imagine a stream that is moving sluggishly. The algae and waste products of the stream begin to build up and clog the system. This is an unhealthful situation. Only by removing the blockage at the outlet of the stream, or increasing the force of its flow, can we reestablish a healthful state. Regular exercise, lasting at least thirty minutes per session, will, similarly, help maintain the flow of your lymphatic system.

2. *Sweating:* The next important goal to accomplish by exercising is to heat the body to the point at which sweating occurs. Viral replication is inhibited by high temperatures. Exercise can decrease viral activity by raising your body temperature to this level.

Sweating serves another function. When the blood vessels of the skin dilate, the sweat glands act as tiny filters to remove toxins and waste products. The waste is then pumped to the surface of the skin as sweat. This cleansing action is very important to the body. It is also important that you shower off after you exercise so that these toxins are not left on the surface of your skin.

3. *Exercise for at least one-half hour:* It is important to improve the circulation to the deeper organs of your body as much as possible. To achieve this, your exercise session must last at least one-half hour. This allows enough time for the flow of blood to extend into the deep tissues of the spleen, liver, kidneys, lymph nodes, and bone marrow, bringing a fresh flow of oxygen and healthful nutrients to these organs.

When you are sedentary, white blood cells begin to stick to the walls of your blood vessels and become dormant. When aerobic exercise is performed, the white blood cells, including T-helper cells and macrophages, awaken and are swept back into the circulation, where they can function at peak efficiency. This process is known as "demargination," and it occurs approximately thirty minutes into an aerobic workout. The benefits that occur as a result of this process will last for hours.

To complement your exercise program, you can add other activities that produce many of the same benefits. These include dry saunas, steam rooms, and hot tubs. They all help to reduce stress, improve circulation, and enhance the body's ability to excrete waste products and can be incorporated into your overall program.

If you feel overly tired or sore the day after you exercise, it is a sign that your session was too strenuous. If you feel invigorated, the intensity level was just right. This rule of thumb also goes for saunas, steam rooms, and hot baths. If you become dizzy or do not feel well when you finish, it was probably too vigorous for your system.

Remember: a powerful and harmonious *combination* of health-promoting activities is the goal of the Comprehensive Healing Program for HIV. Together they will suppress viral activity and enhance the functioning of your immune system. Continue to strive for *balance, moderation,* and *growth* in all of the therapies that make up your program.

Summary

1. Find exercise activities that you *enjoy*.

2. Exercise *three to five times a week* for at least *thirty minutes per session*.

3. Strive to promote *deep breathing* and *sweating*.

STRESS REDUCTION

What Is Stress?

I usually do not enjoy speaking about stress because as the subject is discussed, people usually become tense. This is perfectly understandable. There is so much stress in our lives that it appears that we are becoming obsessed with finding ways to avoid it.

The dictionary defines *stress* as a force, pressure, strain, or weight. These are not the conditions under which maximal healing occurs. Stress encourages just the opposite. It creates an environment that directly impedes healing, regeneration, and growth.

Deep Relaxation

I cannot emphasize enough the importance of regularly practiced deep relaxation. When we relax completely, the baseline activity level of many of our bodily systems decreases. For example, our heart rate slows. Breathing becomes deeper and more regular. All of our muscles relax and utilize less energy. The mind also quiets and consumes less fuel. All of these effects directly contribute to an overall conservation of energy.

Results reported in a 1992 study from the University of Miami Medical School showed that HIV-positive men who practiced regular relaxation techniques or did regular aerobic exercise had higher blood levels of T-helper cells six weeks after hearing the results of their HIV tests than those who did not. Additionally, over a two-year follow-up period, those who continued to practice relaxation and aerobic exercise regularly stayed healthier longer.

The study participants who went on to develop symptoms or die, researchers found, were among the least diligent in practicing the relaxation techniques or aerobic exercise, were most distressed upon learning their diagnosis, and tended to deny the need to take steps to cope with their situation. Researchers say the findings of this study suggest that HIV-positive individuals who are still healthy may benefit emotionally, as well as immunologically, from the regular practice of relaxation techniques and moderate exercise in addition to their other treatments. Dr. Mary Anne Fletcher, director of the Clinical Immunology Lab at the university, stated that the increase observed in the study participants' T-4 cells "was about the same as you would expect in the same period if you gave the patients AZT."

Regularly conserving energy is extremely important to a person who has a chronic infection. If a general energy imbalance is present and persists over a long period of time in the presence of an HIV infection, the immune system will inevitably weaken. It is as if your energy checking account is constantly in the red. Eventually, you will not have any energy left to expend.

Deep relaxation, practiced twice daily, allows your body to conserve energy and work to restore its energy balance. It can also help you create an energy surplus. In order to increase the chances that my patients practice deep relaxation regularly, I provide them with cassette tapes containing pre-recorded relaxation exercises. Each exercise lasts approximately 15–20 minutes and I recommend that one be listened to twice daily. Approximately 15–20 minutes per session is the optimal length of time for a relaxation tape. In this amount of time, its benefit can be achieved without the technique creating stress by taking too much time out of your day. Yoga and meditation are also good techniques that can be practiced regularly to promote deep relaxation.

Conserving your energy for fifteen to twenty minutes twice a day goes a long way to helping your body restore and maintain its energy balance. Energy stored during this time can be channeled toward your immune system. It can then be used by your body to regenerate its cells, repair tissues, rebuild the blood and, in general, shore up your defenses. It is similar to declaring a cease-fire twice daily in the midst of a battle; it allows you to repair equipment, feed the troops, rebuild embankments, and stay at full strength, instead of constantly being worn down by the enemy.

In addition to providing physical benefits, deep relaxation encourages the mind to rest and become quiet. The relaxation tapes that I provide include positive affirmations to help promote a lessening of fear and a strengthening of a positive attitude. The benefits of a positive emotional state are extensive and well worth achieving. They will be discussed in detail in the next chapter on emotional healing.

A second, more demanding, technique for establishing a positive energy balance is called "your healing hour" and can be found in the Specific Techniques section of the Emotional Healing chapter. It is one of the most effective relaxation exercises I know of for helping a person return to balance. You may want to keep this technique in reserve and use it when your T-cells especially need a boost.

Long-Term Stressors

Another important way to reduce stress is by making positive changes in your life that focus on lessening your stress *in the long term*. These may include finding a new job, getting out of an unhealthy relationship (or into a healthy one), learning to establish healthy boundaries in your interactions with other people, or beginning to include a spiritual practice in your life. These activities might be called "making big changes in your life." They have the potential to significantly lessen your stress in the long run.

There is often a substantial amount of fear when it comes to making these changes. This is because a known situation, even if it is an unhealthy one, often feels safer and less frightening than an unknown one. In the next section, I will introduce many techniques that will help you identify the positive changes that need to be made in your life to further your healing. These techniques are also designed to help you overcome any fear that might be holding you back from making these changes.

Honoring Your Illness

Some people say that being diagnosed with a major, life-threatening illness is your spirit's way of communicating the urgent need to make big changes in your life. It might be that you have been depressed and unhappy for so long, without taking any major steps toward improving your situation, that your mind/body/spirit is forced to send you an even stronger message than plain old depression or unhappiness. It sends you a message that it hopes you will now heed; it sends you a physical illness.

The occurrence of a life-threatening physical illness might be the final straw that forces you to stop and reevaluate who you are, what you are doing, where you are going with your life, and whether this is the most healthful or skillful path for you to take. It might finally get you to notice how you have really been feeling.

Psychological distress has often been shown to precede the occurrence of a major physical illness such as a heart attack or cancer. It has also been shown to alter T-cell subsets and depress the overall strength of the immune system. In general, T-helper cells play a crucial role in enhancing the immune system's response to infections, while T-suppressor cells have been shown to do just the opposite. Psychological distress lowers the T-helper cell number and raises the T-suppressor cell number, effectively lowering one's resistance to disease.

The majority of PWAs (people with AIDS) who have survived for greater than five years, as well as most individuals who have achieved complete remissions from serious illnesses such as cancer, have *listened to their body's signals* and made major changes in their previously unhealthful and out-of-balance lifestyles. Making big changes in your life takes you in a direction away from the cause of your stress (such as a bad job, an unhealthy relationship, or a bad living situation) and toward new experiences. At the very least, these new experiences can be invigorating and stimulating. Don't be afraid to make the big changes that you understand, deep inside, you need to make. Who knows? Things could turn out better than you might expect.

Being diagnosed with a major physical illness is not a sign that you are permanently broken. It is not a sign that you are a failure or that you are weak. It is a message from yourself that *now is the time to make these changes.* Change is the only constant in the universe. It is always occurring. Don't be afraid of what the future will hold if you change. Fear it only if you are avoiding change and growth.

Additional examples of how "making big changes in your life" can be beneficial immunologically may be found in the Case Histories: Examples of Viral Dormancy chapter.

I hope that this chapter has not "stressed you out" too much. Instead, my goal has been to provide you with the motivation and confidence necessary to incorporate both deep relaxation and long-term stress reduction into your Comprehensive Healing Program.

Stress Reduction Activities

meditation	exercise	massage
relaxation tape	playing music	hot tub
afternoon nap	mud bath	taking a bath
yoga	reading a book	acupuncture
beach walking	biofeedback	planning a vacation

Summary

1. Keep your stress level as low as possible.

2. Practice deep relaxation twice daily for fifteen to twenty minutes.

3. Make major changes in your life that will lessen your long-term stress.

EMOTIONAL
HEALING

Comes a time . . .
when the blind man takes your hand
and says: "Don't you see?"
You've got to make it somehow . . . on
the dreams you still believe.
Don't give it up . . . you've got an
empty cup.
Only love can fill. Only love can fill.

Robert Hunter

THE IMPORTANCE OF GROWTH

Consider this statement: "If you are not growing, you are just hanging on and waiting to die." What does it mean?

Let us take an example from nature. Consider a plant that is growing next to a riverbed. It is battling many forces that are attempting to wash it away and end its existence. These forces include gravity, the water rushing by it, the elements of cold and wind, and its need for light. If the plant is not *actively* pushing its roots deeper and extending its leaves outward, it will not be able to withstand the forces that are trying to wash it away. If it is not *actively striving* to grow, it will gradually lose ground.

If an HIV-positive individual does not actively strive to achieve growth on all levels—physical, emotional, and spiritual—he may find that the forces of entropy have an edge. One of the fundamental principles of the Comprehensive Healing Program is, *If growth is occurring, the organism will remain healthy and strong.* To stay ahead of opposing forces, the individual must maintain the process of growth.

Once an individual has made positive changes on a physical level, there is an enormous opportunity to continue experiencing growth on other levels as well. By growing emotionally and spiritually, we are able to experience the healing effects that the mind can have on the body.

A large number of researchers are lining up behind the theory that the mind can positively affect the functioning of the immune system. Many recent studies support the belief that your psychological response to illness has the ability to significantly affect your health. The techniques described in the following section enable you to "tap into" the immune-strengthening potential of your mind.

In 1989, Lydia Temoshok, an assistant professor of psychiatry at the University of California, San Francisco, conducted a study on eighteen AIDS patients. It included interviews, blood analyses, and extensive psychological testing. After six weeks, the results showed that higher numbers of white blood cells were correlated with individuals possessing *low levels* of depression and anger.

Another study by Nancy P. Blaney and her colleagues at the University of Miami found that men who easily expressed their anger had better immune-system functioning than men who reacted to hardship with anxiety and loneliness. Focusing on the problem and taking steps to find a possible solution were coping strategies linked to greater natural killer-cell activity and T-lymphocyte response.

Another strategy described by Dr. Blaney was dubbed "positive reinterpretation and growth." This coping mechanism was used by many individuals who were making the best of their situation; they viewed their infection as an opportunity for self-exploration and growth. This was also linked to improved immune-system strength.

The rationale for the above observations was summarized in a 1981 article in the journal *Science,* by Vernon Riley, chairman of the Department of Microbiology, Pacific Northwest Research Foundation. "Emotional, psychosocial and anxiety-stimulated stress produces increased concentrations of adrenal hormones through well-known neuroendocrine pathways. A direct consequence of these increased [adrenal hormone] concentrations is injury to elements of the [immune system], which may leave the subject vulnerable to the action of latent viruses, cancer cells, or other pathological processes that are normally held in check by an otherwise intact [immune system]."

Dr. Riley went on to say that increased concentrations of steroid hormones produced by the adrenal glands in response to negative emotional states (i.e., stress) produced adverse effects on the thymus gland and on thymus-produced T-cells. The studies he reviewed demonstrated that anxiety and stress can be quantitatively induced in lab animals and their consequences can be measured through specific biochemical and cellular markers.

The *adverse* health effects of anxiety, stress, and negative emotional states have been well documented. However, recent studies are now beginning to focus on the ability of *positive* emotional states to *enhance* the functioning of the various components of the immune system. These studies have shown that a positive state of mind and the emotions that are associated with it—hope, contentment, and love—can significantly strengthen your immune system.

Dr. Jeanne Achterberg, a researcher at the University of Texas Health Science Center in Dallas, has observed that a positive mental attitude, a sense of continued hope of becoming well, and a willingness to entertain new ideas about treatment increase a person's chances of recovering from some forms of cancer.

In a related study, Dr. Karl Goodkin, a psychiatrist at Stanford University, recently showed that a positive mental attitude could affect the course of cervical cancer. He and his colleagues demonstrated that a woman's mental attitude toward her future, *when pessimistic,* doubled the likelihood of an increase in the number of cancer cells present. Dr. Goodkin believes that the reverse will also be proven true; that a positive attitude can slow, and in some cases even stop, the growth of cancerous and precancerous cells.

Some of you may doubt the effectiveness of some of the techniques that I am going to mention in this section. That's okay. It is healthy to have a questioning attitude when it comes to new ideas. I can, however, give you the benefit of my experience, the support of a growing body of research, and the observations that I have made during the past five years working closely with hundreds of HIV-positive patients. Enormous benefits can be realized through the utilization of these techniques.

An important point to remember: emotional and psychological healing techniques work best when used in conjunction with natural and standard medical therapies. Whether you are dealing with AIDS, cancer, multiple sclerosis, or chronic fatigue syndrome, psychological healing techniques are most effective when utilized within the framework of a comprehensive healing approach.

How I Came to Appreciate the Benefits of Attitudinal Healing

While the possibility of improving the strength of your immune system solely through diet and other natural therapies exists, I began to notice that some of my patients would follow excellent physical programs and still continue to experience a gradual decline in the strength of their immune systems. When I first noticed it, I began to explore the reasons why this might occur.

I have discovered that there are certain emotional states common to individuals who follow a strong physical program but still continue to experience progressively declining T-cell counts. These emotional states include fear, panic, guilt, job dissatisfaction, and a general sense of stagnation.

When I first began to discuss these issues with my patients, an interesting phenomenon occurred. When patients objectively investigated their feelings, it became apparent that the emotional lives of many of them could benefit from positive change. Among the patients who began to institute these changes, stability and an increase in T-cell counts often occurred.

Based on this new appreciation for the connection between one's emotional health and one's T-cell values, I began to look not only at my patients' compliance with the physical aspects of their healing program but at their emotional and psychospiritual health as well. I gradually began to understand which factors might be responsible for either an increase or a decrease in their T-cell number during any given time interval. After implementing some very specific changes, I watched many of my patients achieve dramatic improvements in their T-helper cell numbers and the overall strength of their immune systems.

Healing Your Emotional Self

I would like to offer you the insights and techniques that I have discovered so that you, too, can experience a healing of the heart. If you desire to begin this journey of self-examination, be prepared for positive changes to occur. Do not be afraid. If you are willing to examine your life and make these important changes, a new awareness of your life's purpose will begin to emerge. This includes a realization that we are all here to learn, grow, and love and an understanding that our experiences provide the basis for this growth to occur.

There is no mystery as to how these techniques work to strengthen the immune system. They provide invigorating and life-affirming emotional stimulation which causes the brain to produce immune-enhancing biochemicals. These biochemicals help to keep the immune system healthy so that you can continue to grow and develop. Growth is the most life-affirming process that exists. If growth is occurring, the organism is becoming stronger. It is stimulated and full of vitality. If you want your immune system to stay strong in the presence of HIV, always continue growing on an emotional level.

I would like to tell you about one patient who improved the

strength of his immune system solely through growth on an emotional level. His name is Jim.

Jim believed that he was doing everything right to stay healthy. He had a very healthful diet, took vitamins and herbs, practiced yoga, and kept his stress level low. However, Jim's T-helper cell count continued to drop lower and lower. Since Jim was doing everything "right" physically, we looked for a conflict on the emotional level.

One important issue gradually became clear. The reason for his continued decline in T-helper cell number was Jim's addiction to having anonymous sexual encounters and the enormous guilt he felt about them. He knew that they were not emotionally healthy. He wanted to stop having them, but he couldn't. These activities were a great source of distress to Jim.

Identifying these encounters as the causative factor for Jim's emotional distress was only half the battle. Just knowing that you are addicted, whether it be to sex, alcohol, or drugs is not the answer. It is only the first step in healing the underlying reasons for that addiction. The healing of an addiction is a process that takes time. It takes work. It takes overcoming fear. It takes beginning to acknowledge and accept your feelings.

After some initial hesitation, Jim began to attend SLAA (Sex and Love Addicts Anonymous) meetings. The first time Jim went to one of these meetings he was more of an observer than a participant. But gradually Jim began to share his feelings with the group. He began to share his experiences, his distress, and his guilt. He began to open his heart and face his fear. After three months of this process, *Jim's T-helper cell count more than doubled.* It went from 150 to over 300. There were *no other changes* in Jim's program during this time. Subsequent tests show that it has now climbed to over 400.

Jim's situation is not unique. I have seen many other patients who have experienced major improvements in their T-helper cell number through work done solely on the emotional level.

It is not easy to document these types of changes as specifically related to emotional growth. It is not as though these individuals took a pill or a new drug for three months and experienced a doubling of their T-cell numbers. In fact, they did *not* take a pill or a new drug, or even change their diets. The only change that occurred was a change in their emotional health. A leap of growth occurred. This process produces a flood of healthy neurotransmitters and biochemicals that flow through their bodies and strengthen their immune systems.

Many people say that T-cell numbers "jump all over the place." Some months they are up and some they are down. This is true. It has also been said that there aren't any particular factors that are responsible for these changes. This is not true. Of course there are reasons for changes in your T-helper cell number. Most researchers, however, have not taken the time to thoroughly investigate this issue. They don't spend extended, relaxed periods of time with their patients exploring what may have been responsible for an increase or decrease in these numbers. *There is always a reason for changes in your T-helper cell number (aside from lab error).*

My experience over the past several years of working with HIV-positive patients has shown me that the most common non-drug reasons for increases in T-cell numbers are an increase in joyfulness, a new passion, a positive lifestyle change, a lessening of stress, an exciting journey, a powerful spiritual experience, and an evolution of negative beliefs into positive ones. The most common reasons for T-cells that decline are too much stress, not enough rest, excessive drug use, poor diet, depression, guilt, unexpressed anger, a sense of stagnation, and an overly pessimistic psychological state.

Jim's experience highlights the fact that work on an emotional level can be one of the most important aspects of healing. Do not underestimate the healing potential of your emotional and psychological growth. You can always regard being HIV-positive as providing an opportunity to help you heal your emotional self. If you are sincere about beginning the process of healing and you continue to experience growth on this level, your healing will begin to manifest itself.

Spiritual Growth

One of the most enlightening aspects of my work with HIV-positive, ARC, and AIDS patients is seeing the remarkable pace at which spiritual growth often occurs. It is somewhat difficult to describe to a layperson the effect that the news of testing HIV-positive has on an otherwise healthy individual at the peak of his or her productivity. Once a person recovers from the initial shock of the news, a new sense of purpose may begin to emerge. This transformation can best be described as a restructuring of one's priorities so as to place nurturing oneself and remaining in balance at the top of the priority list. Nurturing oneself and remaining in balance physically, emotionally, and spiritually allow an individual to live the longest and most productive life span possible with HIV. I would like to describe to you another patient whose HIV status served as a springboard for making great strides in spiritual growth.

Larry was always afraid to be tested. He just assumed that he was positive. Initially, he worked on improving his diet, but Larry felt blocked on other levels. He felt blocked in his ability to give and receive love. It was during this time that Larry came down with his first bout of *Pneumocystis carinii* pneumonia.

Initially, all of Larry's energy was focused on treating the pneumonia conventionally and dealing with the emotional consequences of finding out that he had AIDS. After a period of several months, during which he overcame his pneumonia and regained a stable level of health, he soon began to explore how best to remain healthy and live his life as productively as possible.

Larry was not from this country. He had been brought up in Central America and had left his mother and family to move to the United States at a fairly young age. He had always felt separated from them. Now he was faced with how to tell them that he had AIDS—certainly not an easy thing to do. Larry had never felt comfortable expressing his true feelings to his family. However, he believed deep in his heart that he needed to express the love he felt for his mother and the rest of his family and that he needed their love in return. With this realization, Larry began to exchange information with his family about his condition and about how he believed that he could successfully deal with the situation.

This became a beautiful experience for Larry. His family returned his love and completely supported him. The open expression of love and support between Larry and his family removed a great weight from his heart. He was now happier and filled with more love than ever before. He began to look for new ways to spread the love that was in his heart and to attract additional loving support from his friends.

Larry's experience taught him that when you live your life one day at a time and strive to get as much joy as possible from every moment, each day can be your last without any regrets. Instead, there is peaceful satisfaction, a forgiveness and a sense of tender mercy, for yourself and for everyone you come in contact with that supersedes all other feelings and emotions.

I grant you that this is not an easy state to achieve. Larry used his experience with AIDS to conquer his fear and to help him focus on positivity and love. This made his life easier to deal with despite his diagnosis of AIDS.

In the following section you will find many specific techniques designed to help you continue your growth on an emotional level. I do not recommend that you attempt to practice all of these techniques at once. Although they all may be beneficial, you should first choose the one or two that feel the most comfortable to you and that you think would be worth a try. Later, you may want to work with the others. Used in this fashion, these techniques can help you continue moving forward with your emotional growth and healing.

Trust yourself, don't be afraid to explore new ideas and new feelings, and get ready to begin your healing journey!

SPECIFIC TECHNIQUES

Maintaining a Positive Attitude

Dr. Bernie Siegel, in his best-selling book *Love, Medicine and Miracles* states,

> *Scientific research and my own day-to-day clinical experience have convinced me that the state of the mind changes the state of the body by working through the central nervous*

system, the endocrine system and the immune system. Peace of mind sends the body a 'live' message, while depression, fear, and unresolved conflict give it a 'die' message.

[He continues] *Exceptional patients manifest the will to live in its most potent form. They take charge of their lives even if they were unable to before, and they work hard to achieve health and piece of mind. They do not rely on doctors to take the initiative but rather use them as members of a team, demanding the utmost in technique, resourcefulness, concern, and openmindedness. If they're not satisfied, they change doctors.*

This observation is similar to what I perceive in many of my patients. That is, the exceptional HIV-positive patient is aggressive, confident, open-minded, and willing to work hard to heal on both a physical and emotional level. This commitment and dedication usually translates, on a biochemical level, into a strong, healthy immune system and a prolonged period of viral dormancy.

Other helpful tips for promoting a healing emotional environment include the following:

- Maintain good reasons for living. The more good reasons you have for being here, the greater the chance you will continue to do so.

- Give yourself goals to achieve and remind yourself of them often. An example of how this works is Celia, a twelve-year-old girl with cancer, who wrote down so many goals that she eventually realized there wasn't any time to die. Now she is seventeen, in remission, and picking out a dress for her high school prom.

- Find a purpose for your life. Maybe it's to gain insight into yourself, to do volunteer work, or to help others. As long as it feels right to you, it's fine. Be creative!

- Allow yourself to have some form of work or daily activity that is both stimulating and fulfilling. Find a job that provides you with more than just a paycheck at the end of the week. This is very important.

- Work on improving your relationships with friends, family, and loved ones.

These minisuggestions can help lessen the inertia many of us feel in these areas of our lives. Remember, it's just as important to heal and strengthen your emotional self as it is to heal and strengthen your physical body.

YOUR HEALING HOUR

Take one hour a day to devote to your healing. This exercise is extremely beneficial for increasing your T cells and treating fatigue. It is very potent when practiced regularly.

Don't just read this exercise. You need to practice it as you read.

Begin by lighting a candle and saying this prayer: "May the time I now take bring love and healing to my body, mind, and spirit."

Now lie down and get comfortable. Take a few deep breaths. Allow everything to quiet and to settle. Allow your thoughts to begin having a lot of space between them. When you are ready, place your hands on any part of your body that needs healing. If you are attempting to heal the immune system or an emotional imbalance, place your hands first on your heart and then on any other part of your body that needs your healing touch. Love yourself. Be with yourself. Heal yourself.

Feel your body. Notice any areas of tension, hurt, or pain. Gently . . . just begin to notice them. Make no judgments. Acknowledge the pain's presence. And then, slowly, allow your awareness to move a little closer to this area. As you go, breathe deeply, expanding your abdomen completely, and then your back, and then the front of your chest. Deep breathing is very important. Allow your awareness to come as close to your pain as you feel comfortable, and then just be with it. Just experience the place that exists between pain and no pain, between tension and no tension.

Just sit there, on the boundary of your pain, and be with it for a little while. As it softens, take one small step closer. Just be with it. Be with it for a while longer and continue to breathe deeply. You have nowhere to go, nothing to do, just to be with yourself and your pain. Just give it the attention that it's crying out for. Take a deep breath and relax.

In this way you can create for yourself an environment that is better than any other place you could be. And as you get good at being with the pain in one area of your body, you can allow other parts of your awareness to be with any other part of your body that needs attention. If you've taken ten or fifteen minutes to get this far, you are doing it right. You are doing what is necessary to regain balance, vitality, health, and strength.

One hour each day. Aren't you worth one hour each day? Isn't your healing worth one hour each day? You are definitely worth it. You can create the most potent healing environment possible for yourself during this hour. Many people do not take time just to be with themselves and to ask these questions: What needs to surface? What needs to come up? What do I need to become aware of to heal? These are some of the questions that you must ask yourself if real healing is to occur.

Your healing hour can take place in any environment that you want. You can be watching the ocean or listening to a creek in a forest. It can be day or night. Consider practicing your healing hour in a place that helps you remain comfortable and relaxed, such as a room in your house or spot in your garden without distractions. Work on your healing, one hour each day, every day, and you will begin to make progress.

Now continue practicing your healing hour. Spend the hour "not doing" anything. Notice how your mind will constantly think of things for you "to do" during this time. Just ignore it and allow your body to continue relaxing.

As your healing hour progresses, allow your body to find its own natural positions. As healing occurs, repressed emotional energy that has been stored in your body will begin to surface and be released. This release may occur as a deep, cleansing sigh. Such releases are significant when they occur; they result in a lightening of your overall state and may be looked at as individual steps on your path toward healing.

Remember, you are creating an environment that is the most nurturing possible during this hour. Allow yourself to feel safe, comfortable, and protected. You will not be disturbed. Allow the process to unfold. Allow your natural needs and rhythms to express themselves. Be in touch with your heart and with your body.

If you feel bad while you are doing this, do not be afraid. There is a part of you that is hurt, crying, and in pain—a part of you that needs your love and attention. You can provide this to yourself.

Allow the energy of your feelings to come up and move out of your body. Tell the part of you that is hurting that you love it, care for it, and will do everything in your power to support it. As this process continues, be aware of any areas of your body that are in pain or that need your attention and just be with them, just send love to them.

Continue taking deep breaths. Continue letting everything quiet and settle. Let go of whatever you don't need. Continue to make healing progress toward balance. (Allow fifteen minutes to elapse.)

Isn't it amazing what thoughts you begin to have? Isn't it amazing what you feel in the parts of your body that have been in pain? It may feel like you have been wound up like a spring and are now just beginning to relax. Just notice these things. You have already moved closer toward balance. Now, have the courage to do this every day. You need it and deserve it!

During your healing hour it is very important to make sure that you minimize any disturbances. Disconnect the phone or make sure that your answering machine is turned way down. If anyone you live with asks what you are doing, just tell them that you are doing a healing hour once a day. Then get back to your healing. Do not worry about what they may think; it's what's right *for you.*

Remember, your hands have healing touch. The only thing that you need to do to tap into your own inherent healing potential is to slow down, stop moving, and breathe deeply. Be with yourself and place your hands wherever healing needs to occur. Then just get out of the way and allow your healing to unfold. You have the power of healing touch!

FOLLOW YOUR HEART!

"**J**ust listen to your heart," I said to Robert. Just listen to whatever your heart wants you to do and follow it. "I can't understand how that's going to help me," he said. "I just can't understand how not listening to my mind and just following my heart is going to be of any benefit at all."

Whenever you listen to your heart, you listen to the part of you that is *most interested in your well-being.* Your heart's concern is that you experience joy and love and happiness. It has no other agenda. It is very important to tune into your heart's needs and desires when you are trying to heal. (You may also imagine this technique as tuning into a part of you that is commonly called your intuition.)

"Let's try a simple experiment," I said to Robert. "Whenever you need to make a decision, try to follow your heart's desire. I'll write down a helpful aid on this card."

Robert looked down at the card:

My head says to . . .
My heart says to . . .

He turned the card over. It said: *"Follow my heart!"*

"Let's see how it works," I said. "Tell me something that you need to make a decision about today."

Robert began, "Well, I'm off from work today. I need to decide whether to drive back across the Bay Bridge to my home in Oakland for lunch or to stay here in San Francisco and eat. My head tells me to drive back home to Oakland because it's more practical and less expensive to eat there. But my heart tells me to enjoy myself in San Francisco and spend some time in the city and have lunch here."

"Don't you see how your heart just wants you to experience joy?" I said. "Can you see how your enjoyment of life is its foremost concern? Your heart wants you to enjoy your time in the city rather than get into your car and drive back home. Your heart's interest is that you get the most joy out of every decision that you make."

When you follow your heart's desires, as opposed to what your head tells you to do, you will undoubtedly follow the path that is right for you. Your heart is most interested in your enjoyment of life. Your heart wants you to experience the positive emotions of joy, happiness, and love. Your heart wants you to have experiences that are invigorating and life-affirming. These are the emotions that need to be experienced for healing to occur. Your head, on the other hand, has values and beliefs that were instilled in it by other people. These "old tapes" were usually inserted by parents, peers, teachers, and other authority figures from the past. They may not have had your enjoyment of life as their primary concern. Their agenda and their programming messages can be misleading and less helpful to you now. If you can quiet your mind and follow your heart, no matter how small the decision, you will begin to learn how to follow the path that is right for you. This is your path toward healing.

Following your heart allows you to do the things that are most nurturing for you. It's time to surrender and stop trying to control things with your mind. Just allow your heart to lead you through life. There is no need to be afraid. It is the path that you were meant to follow.

One way to begin practicing this technique is to prepare a card like the one I made for Robert:

My head says to . . .
My heart says to . . .

And on the back of the card: *Follow my heart!*

You must develop confidence in this technique for it to work. Refer to it whenever you have a decision to make to help you tune into your heart's desires. Begin with small decisions. For example, what shall I do this afternoon? Shall I stay home and watch TV or shall I go for a walk in the park? If *your heart* wants to go for a walk in the park, go for a walk in the park. Test it out. See if you are happy that you followed your heart's advice.

Another example: Shall I go to the movies with my friends, or shall I stay home tonight and rest? *Your heart* knows what's best for you and your body. If your heart wants you to stay home and rest, then it's clear that you do not have the surplus of energy necessary to go out to the movies with your friends. Therefore, you need to stay home and rest.

Often it will be helpful to say these sentences aloud to enable you to "tune in" to the desires of first your head and then your heart. Your head's desire can be perceived as coming from your thoughts. Your heart's desire is most often a feeling coming from within. Follow your heart!

If you are interested in healing, it is very important for you to learn how to make these decisions. They help keep you in balance. They enhance your enjoyment of life. They help keep you on the path toward joy, love, and healing. Listen to your heart. It knows what is best for you when it comes to any decision. The more you practice with the small decisions, the more confidence you will have with the big ones.

Robert's comment at the end of our session: "That's radical!"

SUPPORT GROUPS

I facilitate two HIV-positive support groups. Each of these groups meets once a month. They provide a place and a time where group members can let down their defenses and honestly express their feelings. The members of these groups share not only the negative aspects of their situation but the creative approach to living which they all practice as well.

A positive group experience exists, to a major degree, because all of the group members are following the same comprehensive healing approach. It helps when they are also being cared for by a physician who shares this philosophy. This provides everyone in the group with a stronger sense of community, and no time is lost arguing about whose approach is better. In this situation, everyone's approach is basically the same, so time can best be spent on expressing feelings and pursuing emotional growth.

Another positive aspect of our support groups is that they are different from HIV groups where people come to "dump" their problems. When this occurs it can be very stressful to the other participants and does not have a healing effect. Support groups benefit from a finely tuned, complementary blend of individuals sharing friendship and mutual support.

A beneficial aspect of my support groups is that most of the participants are not progressing in their diagnosis or experiencing serious symptoms. This fact allows the participants to acquire confidence in their ability to stay healthy.

The results of an interesting study were released in 1989. At the beginning of this study, eighty-six middle-aged women with metastatic breast cancer were divided into two treatment groups. One group received medical treatment alone, while the other group received medical treatment plus weekly group therapy for one year. The therapy group focused on expressing emotions such as fear, anger, anxiety, and depression and also worked on developing relaxation techniques. By the end of the year, those women attending the support group reported fewer mood swings and a higher sense of "vigor." Ten years later, when the data were reviewed, it was discovered that the women in the support-group component of the study lived almost twice as long as the women without the benefit of support groups.

"I must say that I was quite stunned," reported Dr. David Spiegal of Stanford University to the American Psychiatric Association annual meeting in May of 1989. "My original goal was to design a study that would refute the very hypothesis that I ended up supporting."

Support groups provide an experience that can be strengthening to an individual faced with the hard work of healing. They encourage the expression of feelings and emotions. They help to decrease levels of tension, fatigue, anxiety, and depression, all of which can be weakening to the immune system. Consider participating in a support group to strengthen your healing program for HIV.

POSITIVE AFFIRMATIONS

Your subconscious beliefs play a very important role in determining how your immune system functions. If you can change your negative beliefs to positive ones, you can alter the biochemical messages that your brain sends to the rest of your body and, most importantly, to your immune system.

Negative beliefs are formed by events or statements you have experienced in the past. They may have originally been contributed to by your parents, teachers, relatives, or friends. Now that you are older and have a greater appreciation for your own reality, you can choose to replace these negative beliefs with positive ones that will serve you better throughout your daily life. Working with affirmations can help promote this transformation.

For the most part, our parents were doing the best they could as they raised us. The statements they made usually came from a place of love and a desire to provide for our well-being. But *you* can do a better job at creating a positive belief system. You know yourself, your abilities, and your desires much better than anyone ever will. You know what it is you want out of life and what you need to do to get it. *Eliminate the subconscious fears that are holding you back, and many of the obstacles to achieving your goals will disappear.* These old fears are what prevent many of us from acting decisively to pursue growth.

Affirmations can be used to reprogram the "chatter" of your subconscious from negative and destructive to positive and life-affirming. The first step is to write out a list of your negative beliefs, or the fears that commonly arise to block you during daily life. These may include statements such as the following:

> *"I am not good enough to succeed in life."*
> *"I can't heal; it's too much work."*
> *"I'll never attract enough money to satisfy my needs."*

These negative beliefs, when played loudly over and over in the subconscious, can have a degenerating effect on the immune system. It is important to first identify these negative beliefs before trying to replace them with positive ones.

The next step is to take each negative belief and write a positive response to it that more accurately describes a belief that you would like to have. For example:

Old belief: "I am not good enough to succeed in life."
New belief: "I have what it takes to be happy, successful, and fulfilled in my life."

Old belief: "I can't heal; it's too much work."
New belief: "The potential to heal is inherent in every human being. As long as I have life energy, I can heal. I will make changes one day at a time and I will be successful at each one of them."

Old belief: "I'll never attract enough money to satisfy my needs."
New belief: "I know that the universe will take care of me and provide for all my needs with abundance."

Additional examples:

Old belief: "I am afraid of becoming sick. I am afraid that my T-cell counts are low or that they will go down."
New belief: "I am a healthy human being and my healthy emotions and thoughts will manifest a healthy body. I am not defined by any T-cell number."

Old belief: "I am afraid to express my sexuality. When I feel sexual feelings toward another person, I am afraid that I am dirty or not worthy."
New belief: "It is healthy for me to express my sexuality. Experiencing my sexuality is an expression of the love that is inside of me."

Old belief: "I am afraid to express my feelings. I fear that they are not worthy or that I will be ridiculed for expressing them."

New belief: "It is very healthy to express the way I feel when I feel it. I can always express my feelings as they arise in a gentle and loving manner. It is healthy for me to express my feelings."

As you can see, these new beliefs are positive, spiritually uplifting statements that directly address the negativity of the old belief. Evolving the old belief into a more positive one can help you reprogram your subconscious to feel more deserving of things like good health and an abundance of love in your life. A positive belief system can help you manifest them as part of your reality.

The final step is repetition. Repetition, repetition, repetition, and more repetition. This the way that you learn and integrate positive affirmations. This is the way that you transform and evolve the "negative chatter" of your subconscious. After you have come up with a list of positive beliefs, repeat them over and over again until you know them by heart. Once you know them to this extent, they can begin working for you in wonderfully subtle and transforming ways.

You can practice your affirmations in many ways. You can read them several times a day. You can post them on your mirror so that you see them often. You can record them as part of an affirmations tape and listen to it daily. Be creative. The transforming effect of these affirmations occurs best while utilizing all of the techniques in combination. The more you repeat them, the faster the process of transforming your subconscious belief system can occur.

Another helpful technique is to focus on five affirmations at a time. Write them out every day. Say them several times to yourself. Each week replace one affirmation that you have learned by heart with a new one that you would like to begin integrating. Make the repetition of your affirmations a normal part of your daily practice.

Although working with affirmations can help you to spiritually transform your everyday life, within the Comprehensive Healing Program for HIV they are designed as a tool to help you remove subconscious conflicts that have become obstacles to your healing. Many gay men, people of color, IV drug users, and other individuals who make up the HIV-positive community have been told for the majority of their lives that they are not as good or deserving as everyone else—that they are "deficient" in some way. These are not life-affirming beliefs. Everyone who is HIV-positive must strive to believe in himself or herself as a proud, lovable, and talented individual and contributor to society.

One reason to work with affirmations (even if you don't think you need to) is that sometimes negative beliefs are deep-rooted and not available to your conscious awareness. Just as taking vitamins can provide a beneficial insurance policy to help protect you from a nutritional deficiency, working with affirmations can help provide an insurance policy to protect you against a deficiency of positive beliefs. It can assist you in eliminating deep-seated fear and anxiety.

The situation where intensive affirmation work is most helpful is in the individual who is following all the other aspects of the Comprehensive Healing Program for HIV, feels fine physically, but is watching a gradual decline in his T-helper cells. It is my belief that this can often be traced to fear, panic, and negative beliefs held deep within the subconscious. This situation responds very well to affirmation work.

Wil Garcia, a friend and inspirational spiritual guide, said that our emotions arise when our beliefs interact with reality. If our beliefs maintain that life is hard and filled with suffering, then those beliefs will interact with reality to produce painful and resentful feelings. On the other hand, if our beliefs incorporate trust, hope, and an exploration of our experiences for knowledge and growth, then these beliefs will interact with our reality to produce feelings of positivity, hope and joy.

The following is a list of positive, spiritually uplifting statements (affirmations) that you may choose to incorporate within your new system of beliefs:

"I am connected to the power of the universe."

"I breathe in love and light and exhale fear and darkness."

"I am confident and powerful."

"I am at peace with myself."

"I will listen to my body's guidance throughout my healing journey."

"I listen quietly and trust my body to tell me the truth."

"I imagine myself walking in a heavenly garden where I joyfully pick flowers that brighten my soul. The flowers are my teachers, my books, and my guides. The bouquet I make is my own unique spiritual practice."

"I am willing to listen to the whispers of my life."

"I let go of all limiting beliefs and allow fate to unfold moment by moment."

"What I thought were obstacles, I now see as doorways to new possibilities and new beginnings."

"What I saw as blockages, I now see as opportunities for growth."

"I am confident and hopeful."

"I surround myself with confident, nurturing, and loving people."

"I commit to giving all my needs direct and kind attention."

"I trust that the universe will take care of me with love, mercy, and kindness."

"I will ask the HIV virus what I need to learn from it so that we can make peace and it can gently go to sleep."

"I radiate joy and vibrant health from the deepest core of my being."

"I create pleasing and beneficial job situations which abundantly provide for my needs."

"I love and approve of myself exactly as I am."

"I have the time, patience, and desire to develop meaningful and joyful relationships."

"I take the time to nurture myself."

"I deserve to be loved and admired by all the people who know me."

"All experiences are provided to me so that I may learn and grow."

"Opening my heart helps to heal my body."

"I am bathing my body with warmth, positivity, and love."

"Whatever is causing me pain and discomfort I will explore fully."

"I will explore my pain with love and understanding."

"Sending love toward any situation helps it to heal."

"I give thanks for today. It is complete and unfolds for me in wondrous and miraculous ways."

"I have confidence in myself and in all that I do."

"I surround myself with love, peace, and harmony."

"I trust the universe to provide for all my needs with abundance."

"There is a special place within me that is quiet, beautiful, and peaceful."

"I arrive at this place through quiet time, meditation, and prayer."

"I am comfortable, relaxed, and balanced whenever I am in this place."

"I heal to the greatest extent possible whenever I am in this place."

"I am happy to be me."

"I give thanks to the universe for today."

"I see the magic, the wonder, and the enlightenment in each moment as it unfolds."

"Today is perfect for me."

"I am happiness, gratitude, spontaneity, inspiration, laughter, creativity, prosperity, faith, intuition, love, wisdom, peace, harmony, balance, forgiveness, trust, health, and joy. I am all of these things."

"I love myself fully."

"I am one with all of life. I am safe and comfortable."

"Everything is going to be just fine."

These and other healing affirmations can be found within the following works and publications:

The Color of Light Perry Tilleraas, Haper/Hazelden Publications

You Can Heal Your Life by Louise L. Hay, Hay House

"Healing Meditations" a tape by Wil Garcia and George Melton, produced by Brotherhood Press

Faith

To begin the process of true healing, each of us must make the leap of faith described by French poet Guillaume Apollinaire, who wrote:

Come to the edge,
No, we will fall.

Come to the edge.
No we will fall.

They came to the edge.
He pushed them, and they flew.

LETTERS TO THE VIRUS

Why Write Them?

As you will see in this section, many of my patients have expressed a measure of appreciation that HIV has become a part of their lives. Its presence has helped them begin to make the changes that they have always wanted to make. They eat better, get plenty of rest, meditate or pray, love themselves more fully, and have become more expressive of their feelings and emotions. It has motivated them to nurture themselves and make the positive lifestyle changes necessary for sustained growth.

A good diet, exercise, and a minimum of stress will help you stay balanced *physically*. But as many of my patients have discovered, that is not enough. It is not enough to balance and support only your physical body. It is not enough just to take your vitamins and medications. You must also begin to explore your feelings, your emotions, and the needs of your heart. Whether this is accomplished through meditation, attending church or synagogue, seeing a therapist, or by practicing the techniques described in this book, exploring your emotions is extremely important. We are all here to grow and heal on this level. We are all here to try to open our hearts as much as possible so that we may connect with the love that is deep within us.

HIV becomes a part of the DNA of your cells. That is why it is so difficult to come up with a "cure." Finding a way to make it become and remain dormant is, at present, the most effective strategy. Feelings of calm, joy, satisfaction, forgiveness, and love help to create a peaceful emotional environment that, through the direct action of your brain's neurotransmitters, encourages the immune system to remain strong.

When you write a letter to the HIV virus, you are putting down on paper the way you truly feel about yourself. It is a conscious expression of your thoughts and feelings about your current situation. Nobody knows what will be released until the pen hits the paper and the feelings begin to flow.

The feelings expressed in the letter that HIV writes *back to you* are a reflection of your subconscious beliefs about yourself and your situation. If HIV writes to you that it is going to do everything possible to kill you in a short period of time, then that is what *you believe* will happen. If it writes that it is providing you with an opportunity to learn, heal, and grow and that as long as you continue to explore this path it will remain quiescent and dormant, then these are the beliefs that you hold deep within your subconscious. The goal is that, through a continual dialogue, a more positive belief system will begin to emerge. At the very least, developing a more positive attitude will help alleviate the immune-depressing effects that fear, depression, and anxiety can produce.

Writing Letters

Try this exercise. If you want it to really work for you, you need to actually try it. See what happens. First take a piece of paper and write a letter "to" the HIV virus. Just express all of the thoughts and feelings you have toward it. Stop reading here until you have completed this part. You may want to reread this paragraph if you are not clear on exactly what to do.

Now, notice if you have in any way sent hate, anger, or intense fear to the virus, and therefore to yourself (since it is within you). If you have, try to explore your feelings around this. Then after completing this first letter, write a letter from the virus back to you. How would you feel if you were in its position, if you were forced to live in an environment that was constantly hostile and threatening? Would you want to fight back, possibly to the death, or might some common ground or mutual coexistence agreement be arranged? I know this exercise may sound strange to some of you (especially those who don't live in California!) but go with it . . . give it a try. You are working with your own subconscious beliefs as well as interacting with another living entity, HIV. Whatever this exercise accomplishes, it may help to lessen your feelings of hate, panic, and intense fear, all of which have a depressant effect on the immune system by means of your body's neuroendocrine pathways.

Eventually, try to begin a dialogue with this virus. You can do this in one of two ways. You can write a letter to it and then have it write a letter back on a continual basis (such as once every week or two), or you can get a piece of paper and put a line down the middle. Begin a running dialogue, one sentence or question from you to the virus on the left and one answer or question from the virus back to you on the right, as if you were having a conversation.

Continue these discussions on an ongoing basis. As time goes by, you may begin to see a possible reason for the virus's presence in your life. You will begin to notice how it can help you improve your diet and the food that you put in your body, how it can help you change a stressful job situation, or how it can help you heal unhealthy, codependent relationships. If there is anything that can get you motivated to heal your life and grow, this is it.

The following letters were written by several of my patients who are practicing this technique. Some have written only one set of letters. Others have begun a dialogue that they continually update at regular intervals. I hope their letters provide you with some insight into the insight-generating capabilities of this technique.

MEET ALAN

Age: 33
Occupation: carpenter
Beginning status: asymptomatic HIV-positive, 234 T-helper cells
Present status: asymptomatic HIV-positive, 350 T-helper cells
Time on program: 4.6 years

Alan's Letter to the Virus

Hi Virus:

This is your host communicating with you. As you know, you have caused quite a disruption in my life during the past few years. When I learned of your presence in my body three years ago, I was devastated, frightened, ashamed, and I felt violated. Although these feelings have vacillated quite a bit, and even at times have been discarded, I still cannot say you are an entirely welcome presence in my body.

Alternately, I can no longer say that you have made my life a nightmare or that I hate your existence. On the contrary, you've imposed a greater challenge than I would have otherwise encountered. You have given me the opportunity to look critically at a shallow and nihilistic lifestyle and a cynical belief system. Had I never contracted you, or learned of your presence, I would have probably not had the time for, nor would I have been concerned with, gaining a perspective on what is fundamentally important to me in life and in death. Had I never learned of your presence, had you not taken up residence, my very own self-destructive lifestyle and bankrupt beliefs may have had already accomplished the job you are capable of doing. Ironically, you may have saved my life. Aren't these the things you are here to teach me? I have learned and am continuing to do so. For this I should be grateful, and I am.

Now you must learn from me. I am aware of your presence and can accept that you are now a part of my life. Your survival depends on me as much as it does on you. You must begin to rest as often as possible or you will replicate yourself out of existence, but not without first encountering a long and exhaustive struggle. I don't want to make this sound like a threat—this is reality. It has taken me a long time to learn what I have from you, and to begin to accept what is. Now we must start working together in a symbiotic manner. I am only asking for you to surrender, as I have, so there will be no defeat.

Your host,
Alan

The Virus's Letter to Alan

Alan:

This is what you would probably want to hear from your virus if it could speak to you. "I'm sorry to have imposed, and I'll be quiet and go away." Unfortunately, things are not that simple. The "consciousness" of the HIV in your body becomes more and more similar to your own. So, it's more likely that the virus would say, "I'll be quiet and go away if you will."

So now you know that it is the territorial "I," the "I" that clings to identity and craves comfort, that is suffering. It is the "I" that is the self of conditioned behavior, fear of extinction, and insatiable desire which is the "I" that you oppose in the virus. It is the low-grade anxiety and dissatisfaction that weakens and sickens many of us.

Be quiet and go away? Who and to where? You can't kill life. We are both a part of the same network of electronic impulses. It is only the imperfect self that drops away—the essence continues incalculably and perpetually. So notice what you are at this moment and let it be adequate. Let the state of being, the state of health, the state of malcontent, the state of homeostasis, this amount of time, this amount of sunlight, this amount of food, this job, this house, this life, right now . . . let it be enough. And so will I.

The Virus

MEET GARY

Age: 51

Occupation: musician

Beginning status: asymptomatic HIV-positive, 362 T-helper cells

Present status: asymptomatic HIV-positive, 399 T-helper cells

Time on program: 4.2 years

Gary's Letter to the Virus

My Dear Virus:

With the realization that you are a guest and I am your host, I wish it were so easy to simply write you a letter telling you that you have overstayed your welcome. But obviously this is not a conventional guest/host relationship, so it looks like I'm going to have to deal with a different reality. Apparently, you are here to stay. I've had many guests in my years, but never one that has had such a powerful effect on my life.

I'm trying to analyze my feelings toward you, and I find that it's not an easy thing to do. Since you have the power, so I've been told, to waste me away, I really should hate you. But I have never been able to let myself be consumed by hate. I have always thought of that as a waste of energy. So the alternative is to make something positive out of a potentially negative situation. Herein lies the ambivalence of my feelings toward you.

I have been aware of your taking up residence in my domain for a little over two years now, and I find that with all your worldwide notoriety, you have been directly responsible for making many changes in my life of a very positive nature. Changes that no other influence would probably have been able to produce. So there must be something to the idea of a natural balance—negative energy causing positive change, and probably, vice versa.

I could go on and list the differences in my lifestyle, but we both know what they are. The unexpected part is that these changes, which are attributed to you, have not only added up, but have multiplied into all facets of my life. So, two years ago when I first learned of your presence, I never dreamed I would find myself in a position to look upon you as a positive influence. But, at the risk of hurting your feelings, given the choice, I would still rather never have met up with you. So it appears we will continue our symbiotic relationship. Which makes me wonder—what are you getting out of this?

Yours very truly,
Gary

The Virus's Letter to Gary

Dear Gary:

I appreciate your thoughts and I am not offended by the bluntness of your attitude toward me. I, like millions of other little HIV's floating around, have been the victim of some very bad press, so it's not surprising that we are held in so little regard throughout the world. But it appears to me that if one such as you can see that our negative power can be harnessed and used as a positive force, then our bad reputation is not totally deserved. Granted, with our great power, we have caused an enormous amount of devastation and sadness on the planet, but let's concern ourselves with the personal aspects of our relationship.

I believe that there is a purpose to absolutely every living thing on this planet, and I am no exception. I am aware of my power to "make you or break you." There are times when it doesn't matter to me which way it goes. But I have been with you a lot longer than you think, and I must confess that there is a bonding factor achieved over such a period of time.

I suppose I feel the same ambivalence you feel in our relationship. On one hand, I have the image as well as the personal characteristics, not undeserved, I might add, of an ogre with claws out ready to attack. Then on the other hand, I see my potential as a sort of missionary. It rather gives me a feeling of power when I weigh these two paradoxes, until I realize that whichever way it goes is ultimately not up to me, but is really in your hands. You have the power to determine my fate. It makes me feel almost like a puppet with you pulling on the strings. Not a great thing for my ego. At least I can take heart in the fact that I am, as you have acknowledged, a significant catalyst in your life. I would prefer a larger role, but, the way things are going, I guess that is the best I can expect. We seemed to have learned to coexist. So let's make the best of it.

Thank you for sharing your feelings with me. It's probably good to have some communication.

My best regards,
H.I.Virus

M E E T   F O R R E S T

Age: 44
Occupation: administrative assistant
Beginning status: asymptomatic HIV-positive, 775 T-helper cells
Present status: asymptomatic HIV-positive, 735 T-helper cells
Time on program: 4.2 years

Forrest's Letter to the Virus

My letters to and from my virus are short. Perhaps I can explain.

I don't know that viruses have or do not have consciousness as we humans know it. I presume they are a form of life that are set up to survive and multiply. Therefore a dialogue with such an organism is awkward.

How it got inside of me is really irrelevant. Especially when framed in a simplistic, moralistic, antihomosexual tone.

No one has convinced me that once infected, death—from the effects of the virus—is certain. I do believe that its effects on the human immune system are destructive but I even question that. Is it maybe something else altogether—syphilis, perhaps? Who really knows?

I simply do my best to maintain and improve my physical and emotional self in the context of having had a very dysfunctional family life and living in a very dysfunctional world.

I have not yet given up on life. There are times when I feel the urge to give up. At times I fight the force that pulls me toward hopelessness. My life view is not written down in some Bible created by others or a Bible created by myself. It evolves.

Where does this leave me and the virus?

Sometimes when jogging . . . only when jogging . . . I imagine my immune system components destroying the virus. Not "you" the virus. Just the virus. That is what my immune system is supposed to do. That is what people do: they fight to survive. They use their minds to survive. That's what I do.

So if one accepts the notion of a dialogue—it's short.

Virus: I will survive at all cost.

Me: So will I, AND if you do have intelligence you will figure out that you can only survive if I survive. If I die so do you.

Virus: Ah! But hibernation is no life. I'd rather die. And further, you will spread me throughout the human race because my vehicle of procreation is the human race's very powerful sexual urge.

Me: So it's a battle, then, between you and me.

Virus: Yes.

I don't really buy that dialogue. It bestows intelligence where perhaps none exists. Rather, the virus is probably driven by a force like the sexual urge in humans or something.

I simply do the things that strengthen me and weaken it.

This is all I can come up with right now. See you later.

Forrest

MEET KYLE

Age: 44

Occupation: architect

Beginning status: asymptomatic HIV-positive, 187 T-helper cells

Present status: asymptomatic HIV-positive, 126 T-helper cells

Time on program: 5 years

Kyle's Letter to the Virus

Dear HIV:

My initial emotional response to the task of writing to you is anger and resistance. I am reluctant to honor some creepy little virus by addressing it in letter form—addressing it as "you" as if it understands or responds to logic or even cares. Anyway, here are my thoughts.

My responses to you are confusing and contradictory.

I am, first of all, unwilling to see you as "my" virus or as a cellular part of me. I fiercely maintain my separateness from you. I am revolted at being considered at one with something which brings such pain and suffering. I see you as a mindless invader, but one that I can't even hate because you are mindless and without calculated motive.

Despite the knowledge that healing is love and forgiveness I cannot truthfully say that I love and forgive you with 100% of my being. Despite testimony of those who say that you have been for them an unexpected friend and ultimately a wonderful gift, I can't pretend to be 100% grateful. Despite the knowledge that anger, fear, and negativity are detrimental to me and fuel to you, I can't truthfully say that I've let these emotions go completely.

What I really want is for you to just go away—simple as that. I also want to ignore and avoid dealing with you. These have been my traditional methods of dealing with problems and I feel angry that they aren't working now.

While part of me condemns you, part of me must begrudgingly acknowledge that my life and world have definitely changed because of you. I have learned some things—amongst others:

- I have begun a process of self-exploration long avoided, and strangely enough, I feel excitement and anticipation for the possibilities opening to me.

- I've begun, in the last couple of years, to wonder daily (even hourly) about my purpose here, my gifts to give, and my lessons to be learned. Sometimes I can't think of anything else. I truly feel that the answers to any questions will come from inside rather than an outside source. That is a new concept for me.

- I *know* now that expressing my feelings, opening my heart; letting go of my separateness from the world, and loving and forgiving myself are my healing.

- I know now that healing is an ongoing process and not a final state.

- I'm learning to transform the energy of fear by focusing on love. Best of all, I can actually *feel* it working.

So, maybe I wouldn't have learned these things at this point in my life were I not your "host." Nevertheless, you are an unwelcome guest who seems unwilling to take the hint and go. It remains for me, therefore, to make peace with you—that is my challenge.

Signed,
Kyle

The Virus's Letter to Kyle

Well Kyle—I am here and you can't pretend otherwise. Now you must deal with me.

Do you see me only as a threat? Are you acting or reacting in response to me? Isn't there some way you can benefit?

I've noticed in you, these last two years, panic, fear, depression, and stress. I get from you hostility, avoidance, and contempt. You haven't really been very friendly or hospitable. You haven't asked me what you can learn from me or how I can suggest maintaining a harmonious relationship between us.

If you were to ask, what would I offer as advice? And if I offered, would you listen and trust my answer or suspect deception?

First, I might suggest that you already have the answers to your questions. They are within you.

1. Why am I here? Something about your having to deal with lifelong feelings of separateness from other people—a lesson you've resisted learning. And a lesson of self-love and forgiveness. Also, a lesson of expressing all your feelings.

2. How can you get through times of fear and doubt? Have faith in faith and a power higher than your ego. Let go of thinking that you have to do it all by yourself and simply give yourself love rather than criticism.

3. How can you live peacefully and happily with me? Well, you have been given a talent of visualization which you've used mainly to manifest buildings and objects outside of yourself as an architect. Up to now you haven't applied this ability to your well-being as much as you are able.

4. How long will all this take? Well, get used to the fact that you are involved in a daily process which you simply will take step by step as long as you choose.

Let go of the anger.

Signed,
HIV

MEET JOSEPH

Age: 41
Occupation: waiter
Beginning status: asymptomatic HIV-positive, 248 T-helper cells
Present status: asymptomatic HIV-positive, 234 T-helper cells
Time on program: 4 years

Joseph's Letter to the Virus

Dear V,

Even the idea of composing a letter to you has been a source of dread and anxiety to me for the last several days. The origin of this angst is predicated in the notion that I basically have an unwillingness to acknowledge your presence. The situation is further complicated by my inclination to sublimate my feelings.

My capacity to experience the full spectrum of my feelings has been limited throughout my life. Reviewing my childhood and recognizing the dysfunctional behavior that existed within my family, it makes me aware that I had little guidance in learning how to process my feelings. My family was shell-shocked with repeated marriages and divorces and this resulted in the propensity for family members, including myself, to stuff their feelings and keep secrets from each other. The range of my feelings has never been broad. I hit a switch when a painful memory or feeling arises and, consequently, I seldom feel elation. The quality of my feelings is somewhat homogeneous.

There are some positive and redeeming aspects of our alliance. You have been the catalyst and partial motivator in dealing with my alcoholism and drug addiction. I have a renewed interest in life. In the beginning stages of understanding that we share the same body, you more or less instilled in me a mandate to clean up my act. Your presence was an indicator likened to a yellow flag suggesting that my lifestyle was unhealthy and my behavior less than life supporting.

Knowing you and accepting you to the best of my ability has required a commitment to change. Releasing old behavior is a daily effort. Forming and shaping a new attitude, learning about nutrition, and being willing to grow spiritually and emotionally are ways in which my perception has been modified.

This process of change and growth is often unsettling. I am no longer running away from feelings such as fear, anger, envy, and jealousy (to name a few). This is new for me and is exciting and frightening at the same time. Because of you, I am somewhat motivated, if not forced, to find out who I am and to live and love my life. I also must alleviate the process of sabotaging my feelings and burying myself under layers of bullshit.

I am afraid you and I realize that this fear is a catalyst for change. I don't want to change because of fear. I want it to be an expression of love and acceptance and nurturing. Trying to work at keeping my thoughts conducive to giving and receiving love in a healthy way seems sometimes like an exercise in futility. I sometimes feel that if I do all I can to change, let go and accept, that I'm working the barter system or cutting a deal. Good and noble motives in exchange for good health.

Since there is little likelihood of your exiting from my life, I am willing to do whatever it takes to suppress any harmful effects you might exhibit while residing in my body. I am working toward a love for myself and all that is in my life because love empowers me and renders you innocuous.

Joseph

The Virus's Letter to Joseph

Joseph:

I know that you have great difficulty acknowledging my existence. You feel that, even though I continue to keep from manifesting myself in any overt sign of illness, you still cannot feel comfortable focusing your energy on everything else in your life.

I know you feel extremely well physically. It is good to see that you are truly finding value in your health and that you are learning to love yourself and others as well as learning to accept and let go in life. Before my arrival, your life was unfocused and you were in a process of self-destruction. I have actually been a benefit to you because I have been an integral contributor to making you realize that your life was not working and that changes in perceptions and attitudes were necessary in order to create a more manageable and fulfilling life.

I know that my presence invokes feelings of ambivalence concerning both the present and the future. Some days you feel secure and confident that you will have many more years of flourishing health and well-being. On other days, you are overwhelmed with fear and self-doubt. You wonder about the development of our relationship. You see the havoc that my counterparts have wreaked upon the lives of many that you have known and loved. I realize that when you lose another friend, your confidence is at least temporarily undermined. At these times, you feel that life is a relentless exercise in futility.

Will I remain in this benign state? You don't know the answer to this question. The only thing you have is your life today. Continue to recognize, appreciate, and nurture your life today. It is hard at times to stay in the present, but this is all we have.

HIV

A Dialogue

The following is an example of what can occur when a person writes multiple letters to his virus over time. This is the ultimate goal of the "letters to the virus" technique. It enables individuals to continually check in with their feelings and positively evolve their belief system.

M E E T   J A C K

Age: 46

Occupation: data processing manager

Beginning status: asymptomatic HIV-positive, 525 T-helper cells

Present status: asymptomatic HIV-positive, 604 T-helper cells

Time on program: 4 years

Jack's Letter to the Virus

Dear HIV,

You probably know that I'm pretty angry with you since you're in my body and are affected by my emotions and everything else that I do. My guess is that my anger is another weak spot for you to hammer away at with your insidious effort to kill me. I don't appreciate your attitude and I have *no* intention of letting you progress without a fight. Just because I'm a nice guy doesn't mean that I'm some coward who is going to run and hide from some wimpy little virus that can't even live for a few minutes outside my body. Your best bet is to get out while you still can or learn to live in harmony with me for a long, long time.

As much as I hate you for trying to kill me, I love you for helping me learn to appreciate my life as it has been, is now, and with grace, will be. I have always wanted to live a healthy lifestyle, with lots of exercise, plentiful rest, nutritious food and drink, and meditation, which is for me the gateway to inner peace. Since you've been threatening my life, I have made many difficult changes and I am healthier for my efforts.

Some day, there may be a drug that I can use to stop you from progressively destroying my immune system. But I only have *now* in which to live. So through my efforts, and the support of those who care, I am slowing your progress and perhaps reversing your deadly pattern.

I want to live and you will not find me an easy victim.

Sincerely,
Jack

The Virus's Letter to Jack

Dear Jack,

Thank you for your letter. I'll put it in the file with the rest of my victims who thought they could escape from my grasp. Once I've invaded your body, you're a goner. It is just a matter of time.

Of course, I'll have to admit that I've been with you over five years now and I don't appear to be making much progress. But it usually takes me about twice that long to make you really defenseless against all kinds of common and not-so-common illnesses.

I will also acknowledge that you have a lot of good habits, particularly exercise, that make my goal of killing you harder to achieve. But I'm relentless and I'm taking advantage of your poor dietary habits and the stress you endure to destroy some more T cells.

You offered me the option of leaving your body or living in harmony with you. I reject both. Why should I let you live? My function is to kill and there will be no exceptions. All you *might* be able to do is delay my progress, but you cannot stop me.

So, good luck and nice try but I'll be here waiting for opportunities to further my ultimate purpose . . . killing my victims.

Sincerely,
HIV

Comment: As you can see from Jack's initial letter from HIV to himself, he has a very intense subconscious belief that HIV is an aggressive, angry virus that will kill him regardless of the positive interventions or lifestyle changes that he makes. I pointed out to Jack that these subconscious beliefs create a hostile environment for both the virus and himself which might lead to their eventual fulfillment. Jack agreed that he carried a lot of repressed anger about his HIV-positive status, which might not create a healthy situation. He stated he would try to work through some of these feelings. Jack's next letter, written three months later, is as follows:

Jack's Second Letter to the Virus

Dear HIV,

Just a quick note. I'm working on a more optimistic scenario for our future where we both can survive in harmony. After all, you probably want to survive also.

So let's negotiate a win-win settlement. I'll create a healthy, vibrant environment in my body and you can go into permanent, passive retirement. No more work. Just kick back and take it easy for thirty or forty more years. Please write soon. I'm anxious to know if you're interested.

Jack

The Virus's Second Letter to Jack

Dear Jack,

Sure, why not? It's true that survival is my most important goal and that I won't survive if you die. So, let's give it a go. I'll lay low and enjoy myself by being in remission as you work hard at being as healthy as you can. Both of us can then be around a long, long time. Let's touch base again in about three months and see if our attitude is helping.

HIV

Comment: The following is Jack's most recent correspondence:

Jack's Third Letter to the Virus

Dear HIV,

I haven't written to you for a while but, of course, you are often in my thoughts. Just the other day, I was noticing how the priorities in my life have become more clear. I am also aware of the value of commitment, responsibility, and a willingness to continue living life. At this point, I am happier and healthier due to your presence—a pleasant surprise, considering my original fears about where our relationship was heading.

I appreciate your helping me to value my health more and, as a result, improve the quality of my life.

Our agreement that you remain in remission while I create a healthy body which you can survive in has been mutually beneficial. Thanks for your help.

Jack

The Virus's Third Letter to Jack

Dear Jack,

As you have found out, I am not an aggressive "killer virus" that does not have a dormant state. I am interested in surviving and living as long as possible, just like you. I appreciate the nice healthy body you provide for me to live in. Being in remission is an easy, comfortable state and I'm enjoying it like an "early retirement."

Our agreement is beneficial to both of us and I hope your good health continues to get even better.

Thanks for keeping in touch.

Sincerely,
HIV

Comment: Jack has remained asymptomatic and healthy since adding this technique to his program. His T-helper cells are now higher than they were three years ago. He continues to look for ways to strengthen his program on all levels and believes that a combined physical, emotional, and spiritual approach has been, and will continue to be, essential to his success.

STANDARD
MEDICAL
THERAPIES

Introduction

The intelligent and effective use of standard medical therapies will always play an essential role in the treatment of HIV. Beneficial standard medical therapies include antibiotics for persistent sinus infections, Bactrim or Dapsone as a prophylaxis against *Pneumocystis carinii* pneumonia (PCP), and antiviral medications to treat HIV-related symptoms or a positive P-24 antigen level.

Listed below are four indications for the use of standard medical therapies in the management of HIV:

1. To treat specific symptoms (such as fever, fatigue, and weight loss)

2. To treat specific infections, either minor or opportunistic.

3. If there is a declining trend in your T-helper cell number and it is below 500 cells per cubic millimeter (mm^3).

4. If you have a positive P-24 antigen level.

Standard medical therapies have been used for the treatment of acute infections with excellent results. Infections such as meningitis, toxoplasmosis, cytomegalovirus (CMV), *Mycobacterium avium intracellulare* (MAI), and PCP do not respond well to vitamins and herbal treatments. If you are treating a minor symptom or condition, it is possible to first try natural therapies and then switch to standard medical treatment if it does not improve quickly. For the treatment of more severe symptoms, such as headaches, fever, nausea, or diarrhea, that last for more than three days, this would be unwise. It is important to consult your physician immediately if these occur so that he or she can appropriately evaluate and treat your situation.

Changing Survival Rates

In the mid-1980s, when the first cases of *Pneumocystis* pneumonia hit the nation's hospitals, most patients' chances of survival were so poor that their physicians usually considered not placing them in their hospital's intensive care unit. Since then, both the acute and chronic management of HIV disease and its associated infections has improved dramatically. During the past four years, as reported in the July 1991 issue of the *Journal of the American Medical Association,* almost fifty percent of AIDS patients with *Pneumocystis* pneumonia and its worst complication, respiratory failure requiring temporary ventilator support, went home from the hospital. Thirty-seven percent of this group survived at least an additional year.

The Centers for Disease Control (CDC) has recently released data showing that the median survival rate of individuals after being diagnosed with AIDS (as defined by the occurrence of an opportunistic infection or Kaposi's Sarcoma), has continued to improve throughout the 1990s (see Figures 1 and 2). This is most likely attributable to effective antiviral therapy with AZT, the ability to prevent certain infections, and increased experience of physicians in treating the acute and chronic conditions associated with HIV.

It appears that the time that it takes for the HIV infection to progress from an asymptomatic state to full-blown AIDS also continues to lengthen. Since AIDS was first identified in 1981, experts have steadily increased their estimates of its incubation

---

Figure 1

AIDS MEDIAN SURVIVAL RATE——CDC DATA

Pre-AZT Era   *Median survival:*
(1980–1985)   approximately 11 months
Post-AZT Era (1985–   *Median survival:*
1990)   approximately 22 months

Figure 2

SAN FRANCISCO GENERAL HOSPITAL MEN'S
COHORT STUDY——
SURVIVAL AFTER INITIAL AIDS DIAGNOSIS

Study participants never   *Median survival:*
using AZT   thirteen months
Study participants using   *Median survival:*
AZT   twenty-one months

---

period. Mathematical projections based on eight years of observing thousands of gay men participating in the San Francisco hepatitis B vaccine study have projected that sixteen years after infection with HIV, 43 percent of those infected *will not have progressed to AIDS.* In fact, as we gain more experience using antivirals such as AZT, ddI, and ddC (singly or in combination), we can expect the incubation time from initial exposure to the occurrence of symptoms to lengthen even further.

Another study completed by the San Francisco City Health Department and researchers at the University of California analyzed the course of 114 gay men infected with HIV before 1982. They found that 18 percent had developed AIDS after 5 years, 26 percent after 6 years, and 28 percent after 7 years. Using a mathematical model, it was concluded that at these rates, only half the men will have developed AIDS approximately 11 years after infection. Further review of these statistics suggests that some people may not become ill for more than 30 years after they were initially exposed.

I am convinced that if we combine improving standard medical therapies with the nonpharmacologic treatment recommendations of the Comprehensive Healing Program for HIV, the symptom and death rates that we will shortly see with HIV will be comparable to those seen in hypertension, diabetes, and heart disease. By utilizing this combination approach, I believe that it will soon become possible to attain a relatively dormant viral state and arrest the progression of HIV indefinitely!

LAB TESTS

Once you have tested positive for exposure to HIV, it is important that your initial medical workup include several laboratory tests, which will help determine the current strength of your immune system and your optimal course of action. They include a T-cell panel (including helper cell number, suppressor cell number, and the helper/suppressor ratio), a CBC (complete blood count), a P-24 antigen level, a beta-2 microglobulin level, a sedimentation rate, a basic chemistry panel, and stool samples for ova and parasites.

T-cell panel

The T-cell panel measures the number of T-helper cells and T-suppressor cells, and the ratio of the two in the bloodstream. T-lymphocytes are the kinds of white blood cells that are most commonly destroyed by the HIV infection. When sufficient numbers are present, they are responsible, to a great degree, for protecting you from opportunistic infections.

The information that the T-cell panel provides can be looked at as similar to taking a snapshot of your immune system. It tells you, at the very moment the test is taken, the current strength of this arm of the immune system.

First let us look at *T-helper cells*. The normal range for this lab value, depending on the individual laboratory, is between 400 and 1,800 cells per cubic millimeter (mm^3) of whole blood. It has been my experience that most individuals above a level of 200 helper cells can avoid the occurrence of opportunistic infections if they are following the recommendations of the Comprehensive Healing Program for HIV.

Because the number of T-helper cells can vary widely, any one test result should always be considered in the context of your previous numbers. I have sent *identical samples of blood* to the same lab and received back results that varied by over 50 T-cells. To minimize these variations, your test should be taken at the same lab, and, if possible, at the same time of day. It is also important to get your T-helper cell test done while you are at a stable level of health and not during an acute infection or while you are on antibiotics.

After looking at the T-helper cell number, I next look at the T-suppressor number and the helper/suppressor ratio. This ratio is normally 0.9 or greater in a person who is HIV-negative. It is important to realize that most HIV-positive individuals will have a lower than normal helper/suppressor ratio, even while continuing to remain stable and asymptomatic.

I next look at the T-helper percentage. This value has been shown to vary less from one test to another. Therefore, it is a more stable indicator of whether a person has improved, declined, or remained stable during any given time period. For example, if the percentage of T-helper cells and the helper/suppressor ratio both increase, in spite of a slight decline in the *absolute* T-helper cell number, my interpretation to the patient is that he has improved slightly, or at the very least, remained stable.

It is currently recommended by the FDA that individuals who have under 500 T-helper cells begin antiviral chemotherapy. In a 1989 National Institutes of Health trial using AZT in asymptomatic HIV-positive individuals, three different groups were treated for an average of one year with placebo, AZT 500 mg per day, AZT

1,500 mg per day. The results showed that in asymptomatic individuals with less than 500 T-helper cells, 8.8 percent of those taking placebo progressed to ARC or AIDS compared to 3.7 percent of those taking AZT 500 mg per day. The group taking the higher dose of AZT (1,500 mg per day) experienced no additional benefit but did have significantly increased side effects. While more than twice as many patients progressed to symptoms in the group that was taking placebo, as compared to the group that was on AZT, it is helpful to look at the actual numbers. Only an additional 15 of 428 patients who were taking placebo would, presumably, have been prevented from progressing to a symptomatic state had they been taking AZT.

Does this information mean that all asymptomatic HIV-positive individuals with less than 500 T-helper cells should be taking AZT? I believe that the above information needs to be factored into every individual's personal decision. However, there are other important factors to be considered. It has been my experience that individuals with greater than 200 T-helper cells who are following the Comprehensive Healing Program for HIV can avoid the occurrence of any symptoms or opportunistic infections without AZT. As I have discussed, these are patients who are following an aggressive natural therapies program in addition to eliminating negative health habits such as drug use, cigarette smoking, and so on. Admittedly, this is not the common experience of most other physicians whose patients are not on this type of program. Therefore, most other physicians would say that they see a fair number of opportunistic infections in individuals whose T-helper cells are above 200 cells per mm³ and who are not on AZT. This has not been true of my patients.

It has also been my experience that individuals who follow the Comprehensive Healing Program for HIV can continue to remain healthy and asymptomatic even if their T-helper cell number falls below 200 and often even below 100 cells per mm³. Usually the only medications that my patients are taking at this point are drugs for prophylaxis (prevention) of opportunistic infections and antiviral medications such as AZT, ddC, or ddI. My explanation for why this stable level of health continues indefinitely is that the Comprehensive Healing Program for HIV recommendations are helping to enhance the functioning of the other aspects of the immune system to a level that helps compensate, to some degree, for lower numbers of T-cells.

The analogy I use is as follows. The United States armed forces is made up of the Army, Navy, Air Force, Coast Guard, and Marines, which are similar to the different components of the immune system. If all of a sudden the number of Marines were to begin to dramatically decrease, there would initially be a vulnerability in the U.S. defense system to some specialized forms of attack. After a brief period of time and several emergency strategy sessions, however, I am certain that adjustments could be made to provide for a strong defense even without the presence of an adequate number of Marines. The immune system of an HIV-positive individual who is following the recommendations of the Comprehensive Healing Program for HIV is like the armed forces. The other arms of the immune system are strengthened to a point at which they compensate to a significant degree for a lower number of T-cells. My point is this: *Do not look at your T-helper cell number as the entire picture of your immune system's health.*

Finally, never make any major health decision based on only one T-cell test. The results of one T-cell test, in light of their extreme variability and penchant for error, is not as helpful as observing a trend in several tests over time. Several successive tests can help indicate whether there is a trend in the positive or negative direction. Decisions such as going on AZT, or taking any other medication with a potential for significant side effects, should be made carefully, utilizing several tests and based upon the presence of a positive or negative trend.

P-24 Antigen

The P-24 antigen test detects the level of a component of the HIV virus in the bloodstream. This test is either reported as positive or negative and, if positive, is accompanied by a numerical value ranging from 1 to 600. If the T-cell panel can be looked at as a "snapshot" of the current strength of your immune system, then the P-24 antigen test can be seen as a determination of the amount of "activity" that the infection has.

If the test is reported as negative, it is good news. There have been very few conversions from P-24 negative to P-24 positive in individuals that I have treated with the Comprehensive Healing Program for HIV. Sometimes a positive P-24 antigen has turned to negative with this program. However, if you have a positive P-24 antigen test, I strongly recommend incorporating an antiviral as part of your overall program. The P-24 antigen test can then be repeated at monthly intervals to judge the efficacy of this intervention.

Beta-2 Microglobulin

Beta-2 microglobulin is a protein that is present on the surface of most cells. It is produced at a relatively constant rate in healthy individuals and is released into the bloodstream as a result of normal cellular turnover.

The normal beta-2 microglobulin level usually ranges from 1.5 to 3.0. A study published in the *British Medical Journal* in 1988 showed that of 111 HIV-positive subjects who were studied at San Francisco General Hospital during a three-year period, those with beta-2 microglobulin levels of greater than 5.0 had a 69 percent chance of having an opportunistic infection during the three-year course of the study. Those with beta-2 microglobulin levels of 3.0 to 5.0 had a 33 percent chance, and those with beta-2 microglobulin level of less than 3.0 had only a 12 percent chance of having an opportunistic infection during the three-year study period. This study took place during a period of time when most asymptomatic individuals were routinely not on antiviral therapy.

The researchers who collected these data recommended that the T-helper cell number, the P-24 antigen level, and the beta-2 microglobulin level all be followed as prognostic indicators while monitoring the immune system of an HIV-positive individual. It is therefore best to look at these three tests collectively to determine your level of immune system strength and to help determine the most advisable course of action.

CBC (Complete Blood Count)

The CBC measures red and white blood cell levels. Red blood cells provide oxygen to the body's cells. If the red blood cell count is low, you may feel tired and fatigued. A low red blood cell count can be caused by deficiencies of several nutrients, including iron, vitamin B_{12} and folic acid. Taking a multiple vitamin and mineral supplement (as recommended by this program) can help to prevent the occurrence of these deficiencies.

Anemia can also be secondary to the stress that a chronic disease places on the bone marrow, the organ of the body that produces red and white blood cells. Additionally, it can be caused by drugs such as AZT and antibiotics and by infections that reside in the bone marrow (MAI, tuberculosis, HIV, etc.).

The presence of anemia should be investigated with specific blood tests including serum vitamin B_{12}, serum folic acid, serum iron, a reticulocyte count, serum ferritin, transferrin saturation, serum erythropoietin, and TIBC (total iron binding capacity). Your physician should be able to explain the results of these tests to you and what they indicate in a clear and concise manner.

If a nutritional deficiency is identified, it can be corrected with vitamins and minerals, taken at therapeutic dosages. If the red blood cell count drops extremely low, a transfusion may be necessary to help boost the number of red blood cells in your bloodstream.

The white blood cell count is a general measure of the cells that make up the immune system. T-cells are included in the white blood cell count. The normal white blood cell count is between 3,000 and 10,000 cells per mm^3. If your white blood cell count is significantly below 3,000, your body's ability to fight off infections is diminished. Therefore, it may be necessary to take antibiotics as soon as possible if you develop signs of an infection, such as a cough or fever.

The same nutritional deficiencies that can cause a low red blood cell count may, except for iron, also contribute to a low white blood cell count. These include deficiencies of vitamin B_{12} and folic acid, which can be identified by a blood test.

A white blood cell count elevated above normal can signify the presence of an acute infection, usually of bacterial origin. The high white count occurs because the body is gearing up its defenses and producing extra white blood cells. A full evaluation by your physician, including a physical exam and any necessary laboratory tests, is indicated if your white blood cell count is above normal. Antibiotics may be recommended in this situation by your physician.

Sedimentation Rate

The sedimentation rate, also known as the "sed rate," is a gross indicator of the level of inflammation present in the body at any given time. If there is an active infection or an acute allergic reaction, the sed rate will be elevated. The normal range for the sed rate is 0 to 20. An elevated sed rate can be between approximately 20 and 100. A level of 75 is more worrisome than a level of 25. The sed rate may be elevated solely due to the presence of the HIV infection, or it may be elevated due to other causes such as acute infections, autoimmune diseases, traumatic injuries, or cancer.

If your sed rate is elevated, it should be interpreted along with your other laboratory tests as an indicator of your overall status. An intelligent choice of therapeutic options can then be discussed and the most beneficial course of action can be decided upon.

If the sed rate is less than 50 and there are no symptoms present, I will usually just follow it with a repeat test whenever routine follow-up labs are obtained. The other tests I have already mentioned are usually much more helpful in providing specific information with regard to the status of the immune system. In other words, the sedimentation rate is a very general test.

Basic Chemistry Panel

The basic chemistry usually is made up of a collection of seventeen to twenty-four routine blood tests to determine the concentration of specific compounds in the blood. These usually include your blood sugar, cholesterol, sodium, potassium, chloride, and calcium levels and a measurement of your liver and kidney functions. The most important of these tests are the liver function tests (ALT, AST, GGT, LDH, and total bilirubin) and the kidney function tests (serum creatinine and blood urea nitrogen, or BUN).

The liver function tests reflect the general health of the liver. If the ALT, AST, or GGT is elevated above normal, the liver is in an inflamed condition, which may be called hepatitis, depending on the severity of the inflammation. Hepatitis can be caused by hepatitis viruses (A, B, or C) and by other infections including CMV, MAI, and amoebas. Additionally, it can be a result of exposure of the liver to too many toxins, including alcohol, drugs, and occasionally excessive doses of certain natural substances, such as vitamins and herbs. One important point to remember is that if your liver function tests are elevated, alcohol should be completely avoided.

The kidney function tests included in the basic chemistry panel are serum creatinine and BUN. The levels of these two substances in the bloodstream are normally kept constant by the kidneys. If there is a decrease in the functioning of the kidneys, the level of these two compounds will begin to rise. This is *not* a frequent occurrence in an HIV-positive individual and is more often associated with other conditions such as hypertension and diabetes.

Many medications are excreted by the kidneys. If there is any decrease in your kidney function based on these tests, these medications should be given in lower doses or at longer intervals between doses because they will be retained in your body longer.

Other Screening Tests

The following lab tests can also be helpful.

Toxoplasmosis titer

This test detects antibodies that reveal a previous exposure to the protozoan *Toxoplasma gondii*. This parasite is found in cat excretions and can cause a brain infection with life-threatening neurologic impairment in individuals whose immune systems have been extremely weakened (less than 100 T-helper cells). If the test comes back negative, you have most likely never been exposed. If the test comes back positive, you have been exposed, but as long as you are asymptomatic, your immune system is suppressing the parasite and there is no need for treatment.

Some of the same medications used prophylactically against *Pneumocystis* pneumonia may also prevent toxoplasmosis. These include Septra (Bactrim) and possibly dapsone.

Regardless of this test result, HIV-positive individuals should avoid changing cat litter or, if it is unavoidable, make sure to wear plastic gloves and a surgeon's mask. In rare instances, patients who have tested negative with this blood test have been found to have the toxoplasmosis infection when a biopsy was performed. This shows that the test may not be 100 percent accurate.

Cryptococcal antigen

This test is to detect the presence of a fungal infection that can affect the lymph system and the linings of the brain and spinal cord. It usually produces fever, neck stiffness, and headaches. If this test is positive, it is a sign of the presence an active infection that requires aggressive antifungal treatment.

TB skin test

The incidence of tuberculosis has recently increased in epidemic proportions. Testing positive for HIV greatly increases the rate at which individuals who are exposed to TB actually become affected with the active disease. Obtaining a TB skin test allows an individual to usually determine if he or she has been exposed and is, therefore, a carrier of the disease. If this is the case, then at some point when the immune system is weak, it will erupt into an active case of TB. It is therefore important to identify whether you have been exposed and, if so, to obtain prophylactic treatment.

A simple TB skin test can identify 90 percent of people with T-helper cell counts over 500 who have been exposed to tuberculosis. As counts drop, the test may begin to fail to show a positive skin-test response, and previous exposure to TB can then go unidentified. Some studies have shown an increase in the effectiveness of the TB skin test for those individuals who are also taking antiviral therapy. A positive skin test for TB usually appears as a reddened, raised area at the site of the test approximately forty-eight hours after its placement. If this test is positive, early treatment with an oral antibiotic called isoniazid (INH) should be begun, even in the absence of any symptoms or chest X-ray abnormalities, and continued for a period of nine to twelve months to completely eradicate the infection.

Routine chest X-ray

A routine chest X-ray is a good idea for any individual who has tested HIV-positive. If the chest X-ray is normal, it will establish a baseline film to which future X-rays can be compared in the event that any pulmonary symptoms occur. There are also several lung infections (for example, tuberculosis, histoplasmosis, and coccidioidomycosis) that can exist in a latent phase without producing symptoms but can be seen on a routine chest X-ray.

Routine Follow-up Laboratory Tests

I obtain follow-up laboratory tests every three months for patients who are stable and not on any antiviral medication. This allows me to judge the efficacy of their program at regular intervals. For these patients, the usual quarterly follow-up lab tests include a T-cell panel, a P-24 antigen test, and a beta-2 microglobulin level. For stable patients who are taking medications, such as antivirals, I also include a CBC and a basic chemistry panel. I look at all of these test results *collectively* before making any assessment. If the T-helper cell number has remained stable or has increased, the P-24 antigen is negative, and the beta-2 microglobulin level is less than 3.0, the lab results are stable and no significant change in his or her program is required.

In patients not taking medications, if the T-helper cell number has dropped on at least two successive occasions, even if the P-24 antigen level continues to remain negative, I will usually recommend an antiviral medication as an addition to the program. If the P-24 antigen level is positive, I will always recommend adding an antiviral medication. In the next section, I will cover exactly when and how to use antiviral medications based on your specific T-helper cell number.

Summary

In this section, I have attempted to provide a brief description of the laboratory tests most commonly used to monitor HIV. I hope that this information gives you the ability to more confidently assess and monitor your health status. You and your doctor should *work together* to make the best decisions regarding your health and your treatment program.

The anxiety that some people experience while receiving these results can, in my opinion, be detrimental to their health. That is why I always discuss these lab tests *in person* with the patient and attempt to give them the information in a calm and relaxed fashion. I usually do not discuss these laboratory tests over the phone.

Large rises in T-helper cell numbers indicate one's overall program is working well, while significant declines call for an investigation into the possible causes and an adjustment of your program to help reverse them.

ANTIVIRALS

Because many individuals already possess a significant degree of understanding regarding the use of antiviral medications, I will first present the Comprehensive Healing Program for HIV recommendations and then go on to a more detailed discussion regarding their use.

Antiviral Therapy Recommendations

As I have stated several times, patients following the nonpharmacologic treatment recommendations of the Comprehensive Healing Program for HIV can usually benefit from significantly lower dosages of medications while still achieving the desired positive effects. Lower dosages enable patients to lessen the risk of potentially serious side effects. Since most of the research studies with these medications have been performed on patients who are not following an aggressive natural therapies program, it makes sense that higher dosages of these medications would be necessary to achieve the desired effect.

Another premise for beginning therapy with lower antiviral dosages is to try to achieve clinical stability or improvement at the lowest dosage first. If this result is not achieved within a trial period of two to three months, the dosage can then be increased.

In patients who have begun my program early, there has been a very low incidence of disease progression. Also, as you have seen in the Private Practice Data chapter, very few of my patients have had illnesses such as dementia, wasting syndrome, and lymphoma. I believe that an avoidance of the overutilization of medications combined with the aggressive use of natural therapies is responsible for these results.

In light of the above information, the following treatment algorithm now governs my clinical practice:

- For HIV-positive patients with *T-helper cell counts above 500,* I strongly recommend instituting the Comprehensive Healing Program for HIV nonpharmacologic treatment recommendations with close follow-up of laboratory parameters every 3 to 6 months. I always reinforce the program's recommendations at these follow-up visits.

- If the *T-helper cell count is between 200 and 500* and there is an obvious declining trend based on several laboratory evaluations, I recommend beginning AZT therapy at 100 mg 3 times daily and repeating T-cell testing every three months. This dosage, in combination with the natural therapy recommendations of the program, is often sufficient to stabilize or improve the T-helper cell count in most patients. If the count does not stabilize, I recommend raising the AZT dose to 200 mg 3 times daily.

  Occasionally a patient will have a strong aversion to taking AZT which I believe is in part due to the higher number of side effects reported by patients who initially took the recommended dosage of 1,200 mg per day. While

I believe a trial of 100 mg 3 times daily of AZT is the most favorable initial antiviral dosage, ddI would be my alternate choice for initial therapy.

Based on the initial study results supporting the use of ddI (described later in this section in detail) and my desire to minimize the toxicities associated with these strong medications, I often prescribe ddI on a once daily dosage schedule. When taken once daily, the dose of ddI can be slightly higher than when it is taken twice a day. For example, if the recommended dosage were 200 mg twice daily, but you wanted to take it only once daily, I would recommend taking the 300 mg dosage as a single daily dose. If you weighed less than 140 pounds, I would recommend that you start with 200 mg once daily. You can always increase to the standard dosage regimen of two times per day if stabilization or improvement does not occur.

- If your T-helper cell number is stable and in the 200 to 500 range, *but you have HIV-related symptoms such as fatigue, thrush, fevers, or weight loss,* starting antiviral therapy is indicated. Several studies have shown a significantly increased incidence of disease progression in individuals with these symptoms who are not on antiviral therapy. I would recommend the same starting medications and dosages that I have described above.

- If you are already taking AZT at a dosage of 500 to 600 mg per day, and your T-helper cell count begins to decline, I recommend adding ddI (in the manner described above) or ddC at a dosage of 0.375 to 0.750 mg 3 times a day.

- In patients with *T-helper cell counts below 200* who have never taken significant amounts of AZT in the past, I initially favor instituting ddI therapy (either once or twice daily) in the same dosage that I have listed above. I favor ddI in this group because AZT has been shown to cause more significant side effects in patients with more advanced disease.

I have also had good experience with ddC monotherapy (0.375 to 0.750 milligrams three times daily) in patients with T-helper cell counts below 50 cells per mm³. I believe that ddC monotherapy plus an appropriate prophylaxis regimen (see next chapter on prophylaxis) effectively supports a weakened immune system, protects against opportunistic infections, and does not overwhelm the sensitive overall state of an individual with more advanced disease.

Often, due to side effects or disease progression, it will be necessary to make changes in the antiviral medications that you are taking. This is okay. Your goal should be to adjust your antiviral program at the "right time." I define this as the time at which the medication has lost its antiviral effect but there has not been a loss of T-helper cells that cannot be regained. Specifically, I will usually change an antiviral regimen if there has been a decline in the T-helper cell number on at least two successive lab tests or a clear progression in symptoms.

When the *T-helper cell count falls below 200* (or 250 in individuals who smoke or have a history of respiratory problems), it is important to begin prophylaxing against PCP. At counts below 50, I recommend beginning medications to prophylax against several other opportunistic infections as well. My specific recommendations for prophylaxing against these infections are covered in the next chapter.

AZT

General Information

AZT is not a benign drug. It is a potent chemical that, while inhibiting the replication of HIV, can block your own body's ability to reproduce its cells. In my opinion, the decision to begin its use should be reserved until there is clear evidence of a declining T-helper cell number. AZT should initially be started at the lowest effective dosage (300 milligrams a day) and not increased until a subsequent T-cell test shows the absence of improvement or stability. This strategy enables the medication to add strength to your overall program without the production of unnecessary side effects.

AZT decreases HIV's replication by inhibiting reverse transcriptase, the intracellular enzyme that HIV needs to reproduce itself. However, it does not eliminate the virus from an infected cell. That is why AZT is not a "cure" for AIDS.

AZT is rapidly absorbed from the gastrointestinal tract with peak blood levels occurring within 0.5 to 1.5 hours. When taken with a high-fat meal, the absorption of AZT may be decreased.

Recent Important Studies

In the initial U.S. double-blind study, participants who received the drug for one year were reported to have a 90 percent survival rate. Without any treatment, the one-year survival rate for a group of similar patients was approximately 50 percent.

Another review of 783 AIDS patients at John Hopkins Medical School showed that 86 percent of patients who had survived an episode of PCP who took AZT were alive one year after their infection. Of those PCP survivors who did not take AZT, only 45 percent remained alive after one year.

Physicians at St. Mary's Hospital in London compared two groups of patients who were diagnosed with AIDS between April and December of 1987. Forty-seven took AZT, and sixteen did not. The average survival time was over 24 months for those on AZT, but only 7 months for those who did not take AZT. Several other studies have confirmed that the average survival time for AIDS patients on AZT is approximately 24 months, a twofold improvement over patients who had never taken the drug.

The following factors have a positive influence on the outcome of AZT treatment: initiation of therapy within 90 days of having an opportunistic infection; a hemoglobin level of greater than or equal to 11 grams per deciliter; and a T-helper cell count greater than or equal to 50 cells per cubic millimeter.

Asymptomatic Use

While it is clear that taking AZT within several months after being diagnosed with AIDS may lead to a doubling in survival time, it has only recently been suggested that AZT should be administered much earlier in the course of the infection.

If the 428 placebo-group patients* had taken AZT at 500 mg per day, it is estimated that approximately 15 additional patients would not have had their condition progress. I am sure the patients in the placebo-group were not following anything as rigorous as the Comprehensive Healing Program for HIV. If they had, this study may have had a different outcome. Accordingly, I believe that the small benefit of AZT reported in this study provides only weak evidence supporting its use in asymptomatic HIV-positive individuals with a stable T-helper cell number under 500 cells/mm³. Additional studies comparing AZT use to an aggressive natural therapies program in asymptomatic individuals would provide a very interesting comparison.

When to Start AZT Therapy and How Much To Use

Deciding when to begin AZT therapy, or any other antiviral medication, may be the most important decision that an HIV-positive individual has to make. It is clear, from a multitude of scientific studies performed to date, that once a diagnosis of AIDS has been made (after the occurrence of an opportunistic infection or Kaposi's sarcoma), instituting AZT therapy at 300 to 600 mg per day will greatly improve one's survival time. For asymptomatic individuals with under 500 T-helper cells, the degree of benefit is less clear when compared to the increased risk of both short- and long-term side effects.

If an individual *does not* practice an aggressive natural therapies program, as recommended by this book, then I recommend that antiviral therapy with AZT be initiated as soon as the T-helper cell number drops below 500 cells per cubic millimeter. In this situation, AZT needs to be the central pillar of the treatment program. However, if an individual has between 200 and 500 T-helper cells, is following an aggressive natural therapies program, and *has a T-helper-cell number that remains stable or improves,* I recommend to continue working with a natural therapies program

---

*In the 1989 National Institutes of Health trial testing AZT in asymptomatic HIV-positive individuals (see pages 125–127).

while postponing AZT use for the time being. This strategy will help prevent any negative effects from this drug until it is definitely necessary.

However, if there appears to be a declining trend in the T-helper cell count, I strongly recommend starting AZT therapy at an initial dose of 300 mg per day (100 mg three times a day). I use 300 mg per day as the starting dose because it usually achieves the desired affect of stabilizing or improving the T-helper cell count while also minimizing side effects. There have been a number of research studies that have shown that 300 mg of AZT per day may have similar efficacy to 500 mg per day. If the 300 mg per day does not achieve the desired effect within three months, then increasing the dosage to 500 to 600 mg per day is a perfectly acceptable adjustment.

In summary, please note the following points: (1) lower dosages of strong medications can achieve similar and often enhanced effects when combined with a strong natural therapies program, and (2) beginning therapy with lower dosages of these medications will greatly lessen the occurrence of side effects.

In April of 1990, Dr. Paul Volberding, Director of the AIDS Program at San Francisco General Hospital, stated in BETA, the newsletter of the San Francisco AIDS Foundation, "If the patient is known to have a T-helper cell count that is less than 500 but stable, it is possible that delaying AZT treatment may be an acceptable action."

Short-Term Side Effects

In a study of 282 patients with ARC and AIDS, more than 75 percent of those who received AZT reported at least one side effect. Adverse reactions most commonly reported during the first several weeks of therapy with AZT include headaches, insomnia, nausea, vomiting, abdominal pain, diarrhea, malaise, muscle aches, rash, and fever. The most common of these are an increased incidence of headaches, muscle aches, and nausea. Patients with more advanced HIV disease can be expected to experience greater toxicity.

Although headache, nausea, and malaise are commonly experienced within the first two weeks of beginning AZT therapy, these symptoms generally subside with ongoing treatment. Occasionally they will persist or become severe enough to require a dosage reduction or cessation of therapy. One can also take medications to treat some side effects, including insomnia, muscle aches, headaches, and nausea, so that AZT therapy can be continued. If a rash or fever occurs as a direct result of AZT therapy, it must be discontinued. A life-threatening allergic reaction, known as anaphylaxis, has not been reported.

Long-Term Side Effects

Anemia (a reduction in the number of red blood cells) is the major long-term side effect most often associated with AZT therapy. It is frequently mild, and a reduction in the AZT dose may be all that is required for improvement. In patients with more severe anemia, a genetically engineered hormone (known as erythropoietin) may be used to stimulate red blood cell production. This may decrease or avoid the need for transfusions while still allowing the administration of AZT. Erythropoietin is also known by its brand names, Procrit and Epogen, and is given three to five times a week as a subcutaneous injection (the same way insulin is administered).

There is a subgroup of patients whose bone marrow cannot tolerate even a minimal dose of AZT. A profound anemia occurs, usually accompanied by malaise and other symptoms, with as little as 200 mg of AZT per day. Because of its effect in these patients, AZT therapy must be discontinued and an alternate antiviral medication explored. Patients with advanced HIV disease receiving AZT should have blood counts monitored every several weeks for the first one to three months of therapy and monthly thereafter. In contrast, patients with only mildly symptomatic or asymptomatic HIV infection do not require as frequent laboratory monitoring. After an initial blood count two to three weeks after beginning AZT therapy, blood counts can be monitored every one to three months.

The occurrence of a low white blood cell count (neutropenia) has also been described with AZT therapy and is often the dose-limiting factor in long-term treatment. A decrease in the white blood cell count to below normal can be seen as early as four weeks into therapy but most commonly occurs after several months.

Among patients with less severe HIV infection, the incidence of serious declines in the white blood cell count are relatively low.

In one study among patients with early ARC, only 4 percent developed severe declines in their white blood cell count while receiving 1,200 mg of AZT per day. Among patients with asymptomatic HIV infection, serious decreases in white blood cell count occurred in only 1.8 percent of patients receiving low doses of the drug. Decreases in the white blood cell count that were rated as moderate to severe occurred in approximately 37 percent of patients with advance HIV disease. Initiating therapy with a low dosage of AZT may be helpful at avoiding low white blood cell counts.

In addition to anemia and neutropenia, another long-term side effect worth noting is the possible contribution of AZT therapy to the occurrence of cancer. While the first two are directly related to the drug's activity and mode of action, the possible association with the development of cancer, specifically non-Hodgkin's lymphoma, is less certain but cannot be completely ruled out.

Non-Hodgkin's lymphoma is an overgrowth of lymphocytes, which commonly manifests in an enlarged lymph node. It can also appear as a lesion in nervous tissue such as the brain or spinal cord. This type of cancer is often seen in people with weakened immune systems. It was recognized as an opportunistic infection and associated with AIDS even before the use of AZT. Recently it has become much more common, and it is the third leading opportunistic infection after *Pneumocystis* pneumonia and Kaposi's sarcoma.

A study was performed by the National Cancer Institute between 1985 and 1987 in which researchers tracked 55 patients with ARC or AIDS who were among the first long-term recipients of AZT and discovered that non-Hodgkin's lymphoma developed in 8 of 55 (14.5 percent) of these patients. The average duration of treatment was 24 months. The researchers estimated that the probability of developing lymphoma was 28.6 percent by 30 months and 46.4 percent by 36 months, while on AZT therapy.

Researchers have long cautioned that the use of AZT might predispose patients to developing cancer because AZT interferes with the cell's ability to correctly produce DNA. However, the authors of the above study also suggest that the occurrence of lymphoma may be "an ironic by-product of longer survival times caused by effective antiviral therapy." In other words, the incidence of lymphoma among AIDS patients may increase as they live longer because there is more time for the cancer to emerge. At this point, the contribution of AZT to the development of cancer is a possibility, but it has not been conclusively proven.

AZT Resistance

In 1989, researchers from the University of California, San Diego, reported observing HIV strains that were resistant to AZT. After eighteen to twenty-four months of AZT therapy, a hundredfold increase was observed in the amount of AZT necessary to kill HIV *in the test tube.* Cross-resistance to other antiviral medications, such as ddI and ddC, was not seen. In contrast, viral isolates from patients with asymptomatic or less severe HIV disease who were on AZT therapy, showed slower rates and lower levels of resistance during long-term follow-up. In all cases, resistance to AZT was demonstrated only in the test tube. It was not linked to a deterioration in the patient's health. Further studies are needed to determine if AZT resistance in the test tube correlates with the clinical decline of patients who take it for several years.

Most recently, results have been released from a 1992 study showing a beneficial clinical effect associated with switching from AZT to ddI therapy in patients who had been taking AZT for at least four months. The group which switched antivirals experienced clear benefit in avoiding disease progression when compared to those continuing on AZT. These results suggest that as soon as a declining trend in your immune status is detected, rotating to a different antiviral may be beneficial.

DDI

General Information

Didanosine (ddI) and AZT belong to a group of antivirals known as nucleoside analogues. Early in 1988, the government licensed the Bristol-Meyers Company to begin testing the drug's safety in ninety AIDS patients. By early 1989, rumors about the beneficial effects of ddI had spread throughout the AIDS community, and hundreds were seeking the drug by any means. In autumn of 1989,

Figure 3

BENEFITS ASSOCIATED WITH AZT THERAPY
(Reprinted from *AIDS Clinical Review,* 1991, Dekker Publishing.)

prolonged survival	increased T-helper cell numbers (temporary)
decreased frequency and severity of opportunistic infections	increased T-suppressor cell numbers
delayed progression to ARC	increased skin-test reactivity
delayed progression to AIDS	decreased serum HIV P-24 antigen level
weight gain	delayed development of positive P-24 antigen
improved performance status	decreased plasma levels of HIV
improved cognitive-neurologic function	increased platelet counts

the government relented to public pressure and allowed Bristol-Meyers to distribute ddI free of charge to AIDS patients who could not tolerate AZT. This was known as the ddI expanded access program.

While taking AZT, AIDS patients have an 80 percent survival rate at 12 months. However, there is a rapid progression of the disease between 12 and 24 months with only a 50 percent survival rate at 21 months. This decline is possibly related to the development of strains of the virus that are resistant to AZT. It would be extremely helpful to have a secondary drug to use, either to prevent this problem or to take once AZT resistance is suspected. It is hoped that the addition of ddI to the antivirals arsenal will enable patients and their physicians to more effectively manage the potential problem of antiviral drug resistance.

Figure 4

POTENTIAL SIDE EFFECTS DUE TO AZT THERAPY

headache	nausea
muscle pain	vomiting
decreased red blood cell count	rash
decreased white blood cell count	insomnia
changes in energy level	fever
liver inflammation	drug resistance

Side Effects

One of the major advantages of ddI over AZT is that it does not usually cause significant anemia or neutropenia (low white blood cell counts) as a side effect. However, ddI does have other significant side effects that must be considered when deciding whether or not to begin taking this drug. As of June 19, 1991, the total number of patients enrolled in ddI research studies was 29,496. The following are the most commonly reported side effects from these studies:

1. *Gastrointestinal side effects* represent the most common adverse reactions to ddI. They are responsible for approximately 20 percent of all reported side effects. Pancreatitis remains the single most commonly reported serious side effect. It has been seen in 2.3 percent of all patients ever enrolled in a ddI study. Early detection and management greatly influences the prognosis of this complication, and it is reversible in most instances. The onset of abdominal pain, with or without nausea and vomiting, should alert the patient and physician to the possible presence of pancreatitis. In some patients, the symptoms can be rather sudden in onset, so they should be reported to the physician immediately. There have been 67 deaths due to pancreatitis out of the more than 29,000 patients who have enrolled in ddI trials. Patients receiving ddI

should avoid alcohol as well as other drugs that may cause pancreatitis, including intravenous pentamidine.

The next most common gastrointestinal side effect due to ddI is diarrhea, followed by nausea and vomiting, abdominal pain, and increased serum amylase levels. A number of cases of salivary-gland enlargement and dry mouth, with or without pain, have also been described.

2. *Nervous system side effects* are the second most common side effect reported with ddI therapy. Seizures occurred in 1.4 percent of the patients enrolled in ddI studies. HIV-related conditions, as opposed to the drug, were clearly responsible for many of these seizures. Neuropathy, confusion, and headache have also been reported as side effects of ddI and are reversible when detected early. After resolution of these symptoms, patients can often tolerate restarting ddI at a reduced dose.

3. *Other side effects* reported with ddI include abnormal liver function tests, allergic reactions, and electrolyte (sodium, potassium, and magnesium) abnormalities. These side effects are usually reversible by suspending ddI ingestion and may not return if ddI is resumed at a lower dose. This is not true of allergic reactions, which indicate that a person is intolerant to ddI at any dosage.

Recent Important Studies

The results of the first long-term study using ddI were reported in the September 1991 issue of the medical journal *Lancet*. The study followed 58 HIV-positive patients, 22 with AIDS and 36 with ARC. The participants took ddI for up to 21 months. Patients who had not previously used AZT showed an average T-helper cell increase of 30 percent after 1 year. Those who had used AZT for 4 months or more showed little or no T-helper cell increase, although they generally remained healthy.

The 13 patients who received treatment at the lower dosage of ddI (3.2 to 9.6 mg/kg/day) had a mean T-helper cell count increase of 50 percent after nine months of treatment. Of the 6 patients with detectable P-24 antigen levels, 3 had a conversion to a negative P-24 antigen level 15 months after beginning ddI therapy, and none developed new positive P-24 antigen levels. The improvement in T-helper cell count and P-24 antigen level continued for some patients for up to 15 months, and the patients who received AZT for 4 months or less prior to starting ddI had greater increases in their T-helper cell counts than those who had received AZT for more than 4 months prior to beginning ddI.

Additionally, 4 patients who had problems with memory, attention, or concentration due to their HIV disease improved after 6 to 12 weeks on ddI, as measured by neuropsychometric testing. This information provides evidence that ddI crosses the blood-brain barrier and delivers antiviral therapy to the central nervous system.

The most encouraging piece of information in the *Lancet* study was the 88 percent overall survival rate after 21 months of ddI therapy. This compares with a 50 percent survival rate after 21 months among similar groups of patients in the early trials of AZT and a 25 percent survival rate after 21 months among those who have received no treatment.

Two additional phase-one studies were published during 1990 in the *New England Journal of Medicine.* In one study, 17 patients with AIDS and 20 patients with ARC were treated twice daily with ddI. The duration of treatment ranged from 2 to 44 weeks. The administration of ddI was associated with statistically significant decreases in P-24 antigen levels and increases in T-helper cell numbers at between 2 and 20 weeks of therapy. In the second study, 17 patients with AIDS and 17 with ARC were treated with a single daily dose of ddI. The ddI treatment group showed an average 57-cell increase in the T-helper cell number 10 weeks into treatment. P-24 antigen levels decreased by at least 50 percent in 14 of 19 patients.

Most recently, an interim evaluation of ACTG 116-B/117 (an AIDS Clinical Trials Group study) in April of 1992 showed that ddI appears to be more efficacious than AZT in delaying the occurrence of new AIDS-defining infections, and death, in individuals who previously had been on AZT for at least 16 weeks.

T-helper cell counts were also higher over time in both ddI dosage groups (200 or 300 mg twice a day) compared to AZT (by about 10 cells per mm^3) but there was no difference in overall survival time. The information from this study tells us that asymptomatic HIV-positive or ARC patients who have been on AZT for at least 16 weeks may benefit by switching to ddI. In addition, the study showed that the lower dose of ddI (200 mg twice a day) is the dose that appears to give patients the greater benefit and a lesser frequency of side effects. This study is continuing.

Dosage Information

In the expanded access program, ddI was available as a powder in packets of 250-mg and 375-mg strengths. The packets contained both ddI and a citrate-phosphate buffer that improved the drug's absorption. Dosage instructions specified that the contents of one packet should be poured into a container with four ounces of water, stirred for two to three minutes, and taken on an empty stomach (at least one-half hour before or two hours after meals) twice daily.

Recently, ddI has been released as chewable tablets. Two tablets must be chewed and swallowed at each dosage interval for the correct amount of buffer to be ingested, insuring that the stomach's acid environment is neutralized in order for ddI to be adequately absorbed. The chewable tablets should also be taken on an empty stomach. Dosage strengths of 100-mg tablets (two tablets equal 200 mg) and 150-mg tablets (two tablets equal 300 mg) now replace the 250-mg and 375-mg strengths respectively.

While Bristol-Meyers recommends that ddI be administered twice daily, the aforementioned *New England Journal of Medicine* study treated patients with once-daily ddI at several different dosages. It appeared that the incidence of peripheral neuropathy and pancreatitis were significantly decreased at this dosing frequency compared with prior studies that tested twice-daily dosing of this medication. In fact, of the 11 patients who had mild peripheral neuropathy before initiating ddI therapy, 8 reported a resolution of their neuropathy while taking ddI at the once-daily dosage. Dr. T. P. Cooley and his coworkers concluded that "ddI given once daily results in improved immunologic and virologic measurements in patients with AIDS and ARC."

I often advise my patients to start ddI with once-daily dosing to observe how it is initially tolerated. When they take it once a day, I frequently observe improvement in their T-helper-cell number and a decline in the P-24 antigen without the occurrence of significant side effects. If this positive trend continues, there is little reason to increase the dosage of ddI or advance it to twice a day. However, as with AZT, if significant stability or improvement does not occur at a low dosage or on a once-daily schedule, I increase the amount of ddI taken at each dose or change the dosing to twice daily to achieve the treatment objectives. Because my patients are also following the nonpharmacologic treatment recommendations of the Comprehensive Healing Program for HIV, they respond much better to gentle doses of antiviral medication and experience significant benefit with fewer side effects. The dosage of a medication can always be increased if significant stability or improvement do not occur. In contrast, too high an initial drug dosage can cause great discomfort and painful side effects in individuals who are very sensitive to a potent medication.

One additional point to mention: In the studies testing a once-daily dosage of ddI, it was found that the maximum amount of ddI tolerated per dose, when taken once daily, was almost twice the amount of ddI tolerated per dose in the studies prescribing ddI twice daily. Therefore, if ddI is taken once daily, it can be taken each time at a higher dosage than if it is prescribed twice a day. Of course you should not adjust the dosage of any medication you are taking without first consulting your physician.

DDC

General Information

Dideoxycytodine (ddC) is the third member of the family of antiviral medications that includes ddI and AZT. In the test tube, ddC exhibits an extremely potent anti-HIV effect. Unfortunately, high doses of ddC used as a single agent in early studies produced painful peripheral neuropathy that often precipitated the need to discontinue its use. More recent studies, utilizing lower dosages or its use in combination with other antivirals, showed a significant reduction of this side effect.

The drug was originally released in an expanded access program by the drug's manufacturer, Hoffmann-LaRoche. It was finally approved by the FDA, for use in combination with AZT, in the spring of 1992.

Recent Important Studies

In mid-1991, the results of several important clinical trials utilizing ddC versus AZT were released. The first study, sponsored by the federally funded AIDS Clinical Trials Group (ACTG 114), treated 600 patients with either AZT or ddC for an average of 19 weeks. These patients had never used AZT or had taken it previously for less than three months. In this study group, there was *no significant difference in survival between the patients taking ddC and AZT*. It was also notable that more opportunistic infections and cancers occurred in the patients taking ddC than in the patients taking AZT.

Additionally, patients on ddC with T-helper cell counts lower than 100 had no increase in their counts. Those with T-helper cell counts over 100 had only a minimal rise.

Neither drug produced a significant effect on P-24 antigen levels. It is important to note, once again, that this unimpressive performance came in a patient group that *had never taken AZT before or had only begun it in the recent past.*

Another study compared ddC to AZT in 102 patients with AIDS or ARC *who had previously used AZT for at least one year.* Patients were treated with either ddC or AZT for an average of 16 weeks. In contrast to the above study, early analysis of this data shows a trend toward fewer opportunistic infections and cancers in patients taking ddC. This trend may suggest that ddC is more effective as a second-line therapy for people who have already been on AZT for more than a year.

The events that ultimately led to the FDA approval of ddC for use in combination with AZT were brought about by two separate studies. The first of these was a study designed to test whether this combination of antivirals posed any risk to patients from unexpected toxicities. Not only was no such risk found, but the combination of these drugs unexpectedly showed a much greater rise in T-cells than previously seen with any single antiviral treatment. This was especially surprising in view of the fact that the participants started with very low T-helper cell counts (a median of about 70). The results of this study were eventually published in the *Annals of Internal Medicine* in January of 1992.

The second study supporting AZT/ddC combination therapy looked at groups of 50 patients receiving AZT alone, AZT plus ddC, or AZT plus ddI (ACTG 106). Although this study is still ongoing, the most recent data released shows a larger rise in the T-helper cell number from AZT and ddC in combination than from AZT alone. (The AZT/ddI combination data has not yet been released.)

The results described in the above studies led the FDA to release ddC in mid-1992 under its "accelerated approval" program, which allows a potentially useful drug to be released after a minimum of positive data has been accumulated with the stipulation that the drug may be withdrawn from the market if clinical benefit is not eventually shown to occur.

The drug was therefore released (brand name HIVID) to be used in combination with AZT for the management of HIV-infected adults with AIDS or advanced HIV disease and T-helper cell counts less than or equal to 300 cells per mm^3.

Side Effects

The major side effect associated with ddC is peripheral neuropathy, predominately involving the lower extremities. Peripheral neuropathy is characterized by a burning pain in the feet that can be accompanied by shooting pains and cramping. Symptoms may be subtle at the onset. Prompt discontinuation of ddC should result in rapid resolution of these symptoms in patients receiving low doses of the drug. In some patients, symptoms may worsen for several weeks after discontinuing ddC before improvement is seen. This side effect was observed in almost all of the patients taking ddC during its early trials at high doses. The lower dosages currently being prescribed (.375 to .75 mg every 8 hours) show a decrease in the incidence and severity of this side effect.

Roche Pharmaceuticals has warned physicians to be aware of possible adverse effects when combining ddC with several other commonly used medications. It is recommended that patients needing radiation therapy, amphotericin B, pyrimethamine, sulfadiazine, I.V. Bactrim or Septra, DHPG, I.V. pentamidine, and acyclovir be extremely cautious when combining these drugs with ddC due to the possible potentiation of its side effects.

Other, less common side effects from ddC include skin eruptions, oral ulcers, esophageal ulcers, elevated liver enzymes, and low platelet counts. Rare side effects that have occurred in isolated cases include fever, hearing loss, kidney failure, and abdominal pain.

Patients participating in the AIDS Clinical Trials Group studies had to discontinue ddC therapy for many of the side effects mentioned above. Treatment discontinuation was most often precipitated by the occurrence of peripheral neuropathy. Oral ulcers, anemia, neutropenia, low platelet counts, and elevated liver enzymes necessitated discontinuation of the drug less frequently.

Combination Therapy

There are several potential advantages to utilizing combination antiviral therapy. First, it could allow an individual to use lower dosages of more than one drug, possibly minimizing the occurrence of side effects. Second, the development of viral resistance may be delayed if several drugs are taken together or if the antiviral medications are varied on a regular basis (every few months).

Early data indicate that ddC and AZT taken together have produced sustained increases in T-helper cell counts better than AZT or ddC alone. The dosages that have been studied are .75 mg of ddC and 200 mg of AZT, both taken three times daily. At present, this should be considered high-dose combination therapy. If an individual is following the Comprehensive Healing Program for HIV and would like to begin "gentle" combination antiviral therapy, I would recommend starting with AZT 100 mg three times daily combined with ddC .375 mg three times daily. The dosages of both of these medications can be increased if stability or improvement is not initially achieved.

The aforementioned 1992 *Annals of Internal Medicine* article on combination antiviral therapy with AZT and ddC was designed to evaluate the toxicity and effectiveness of combining these two drugs in patients with advanced HIV disease. Involved in the trial were 56 patients, 27 with AIDS and 29 with advanced ARC. The mean T-helper cell count of the study group was 65 cells per mm³. None had previously been on antiviral therapy. The mean length of follow-up was 40 weeks. There were several dosage combinations tested and all were relatively well tolerated. Two patients had severe peripheral neuropathy, which resolved when the drugs were discontinued.

At the lowest combination dosage, there was an increase in the T-helper cell count of approximately 30 cells with a rapid decline after 12 to 16 weeks. Using higher dosages, there was a maximal increase of up to 120 cells, somewhat higher than what would be expected with AZT therapy alone. This increase tended to persist for up to a year. As a result of this study's data, the following dosage of the two drugs was chosen for the presently ongoing phase three trial: AZT 200 mg three times a day and ddC 0.03 mg per kg three times a day. For a 150-pound individual, this would translate as 0.68 mg of ddC taken three times a day. Since ddC is available only in 0.375-mg capsules, 2 capsules (0.75 mg) taken three times daily would be the recommended dose based on the above study data.

There is also an ongoing phase-one trial investigating the safety and efficacy of combining AZT and ddI. Preliminary data suggest that this combination is well tolerated and that T-helper cell counts have increased with all of the dosages studied. Individuals in this study have T-helper cell counts less than 400 and have been on AZT for less than 3 months prior to entering the study. Fifty-two participants have been enrolled in varying treatment groups. Speaking at the Seventh International AIDS Conference, Dr. Ann Collier from the University of Washington in Seattle noted that after 24 weeks of therapy, there were no unexpected toxicities and no adverse interactions between the two drugs. She also stated that it appeared that patients who were receiving 600 mg of AZT in combination with 350 to 500 mg of ddI per day (in the powdered form) continued to show sustained increases of T-helper cell numbers beyond 12 weeks of therapy. Dr. Collier noted that too few subjects have had a sufficient duration of therapy to determine whether the disparity found at different dosages will persist.

Long-term follow-up is necessary to evaluate which combination regimen will provide the greatest extended benefits. However, it is clear that a combination of antiviral medications can initiate rises in the T-helper-cell number without excessive toxicities. My recommendation to most patients is that they begin antiviral therapy with a single agent and then add a second drug if there is clear evidence of a declining trend in their T-helper cell number. Please refer to the Comprehensive Healing Program Antiviral Therapy Recommendations at the beginning of this section (p. 134) for specific information on when to add antiviral medications to your program based on your exact T-helper cell number.

PROPHYLAXIS

Opportunistic infections are the major cause of morbidity and mortality due to HIV. By regularly monitoring your T-helper cell count, you can determine when it is most appropriate to begin taking the prophylactic medications that can help prevent these infections. By constructing an intelligent prophylaxis program, one can continue to remain healthy and free from these infections for an extended period of time, despite low T-helper cell numbers.

The ideal prophylaxis program prevents opportunistic infections and is well tolerated over an extended period of time. It should also be acceptable to the patient, be cost-effective, and, if possible, utilize drugs that have activity against more than one type of infection.

The best prophylaxis protocol is one linked to a strong overall strategy directed at suppressing the primary HIV infection. A strategy based solely on preventing opportunistic infections is ultimately doomed to fail, as the success of every prophylaxis regimen depends to some extent on the overall strength of the immune system.

Because many individuals are already familiar with the most commonly prescribed prophylactic medications, I will first present my recommendations in the table below and then give the rationale for their use in the pages that follow.

Recommendations For Opportunistic Infection Prophylaxis

T-HELPER CELL NUMBER	INFECTION	PROPHYLAXIS
Less than 200	PCP	Aerosol pentamidine 300 mg once monthly *or* TMP-SMX 1 double strength tab 3 times a week *or* Dapsone 100 mg three times a week
Less than 100	PCP	TMP-SMX 1 double strength tab daily *or* Dapsone 100 mg daily
Less than 50	PCP	TMP-SMX 1 double strength tab daily *or* Dapsone 100 mg daily *plus:* Aerosol pentamidine 300 mg every other month
	Toxoplasma	TMP-SMX 1 double strength tab daily *or* Dapsone 100 mg daily *continued*

MAI	clarithromycin 500 mg three times/ week *or* azithromycin 250 mg three times/ week *or* rifabutin 300 mg daily
Fungal	Fluconizole 100 mg three times/ week
CMV	None currently available. High dose acyclovir may impart some degree of protection. Quarterly evaluation with an experienced ophthalmologist is extremely important.

PCP (Pneumocystis Carinii Pneumonia) Prophylaxis

PCP is the most frequently occurring opportunistic infection in HIV-positive individuals. In the United States, 60 percent to 85 percent of HIV-positive individuals will ultimately contract PCP at some point in the course of their disease. It is also the single most common cause of death in persons with AIDS. Unfortunately, when an opportunistic infection such as PCP occurs, it also triggers a major stimulation of the immune system, further potentiating the activity of HIV itself. Postponing an initial occurrence of PCP indefinitely is, therefore, of great benefit to an HIV-positive individual.

The T-helper cell number at which primary prophylaxis against PCP is most commonly implemented ranges between 200 and 300 helper cells, depending on the physician or the study that is referenced. In my practice, I begin PCP prophylaxis when the T-helper cell count falls below 200 cells/mm³. If there is a significant reason to suspect a weakness of the respiratory system, such as a prior history of pneumonia or in an individual who smokes, I begin PCP prophylaxis when the T-helper cell number falls below 250 cells/mm³.

The three most common PCP prophylaxis regimens currently in use are listed below:

Aerosol Pentamadine (AP)

Several large studies of AP have been published showing a clear benefit at preventing PCP when compared to placebo. The San Francisco Community Consortium study, reported in the 1990 *New England Journal of Medicine,* showed the superiority of a 300 mg monthly dose of aerosol pentamidine in preventing PCP, when compared to other dosage regimens. This study included 408 HIV-positive individuals and looked at the prevention of both primary (first episode), as well as secondary PCP. The average time the participants were on the study was 7.6 months.

After this study was published, a monthly dose of 300 mg of aerosol pentamidine became the community standard as the prophylactic regimen for preventing PCP.

Side effects reported with AP include cough and wheezing in 1 to 2 percent of the treatments. While these are the most frequent adverse effects, less than one in a hundred patients needs to discontinue their treatments due to them.

Other drawbacks to consider with the AP regimen are: 1) a PCP prevention rate of only 70 to 90 percent after one year of use 2) the rare occurrence of pneumocystis infection outside of the lung, and 3) the occurrence of pneumocystis in areas of the lungs that do not receive adequate amounts of the aerosolized medication. The chance of this occurring can be lessened by inhaling the AP in a reclining position.

Trimethoprim-Sulfamethoxazole (TMP-SMX)

Based on clinical experience and several recently published studies, TMP-SMX has become the most commonly utilized medication for the prevention of PCP. This compound is also referred to by its brand names, Bactrim and Septra. Multiple open trials and retrospective reviews have demonstrated that it is effective at preventing PCP in patients who have previously had an episode, as well as in those patients with less than 200 T-helper cells who have never before had PCP. Because of its low cost, and the fact that it can be taken in pill form at home, many physicians are recommending TMP-SMX as the sole drug to prophylax against PCP. The most common regimens currently used are one double-strength tablet daily, one double-strength tablet every other day and one double-strength tablet three times a week. All of these dosage regimens have been reported effective in recent trials. There is currently ongoing a national multicenter study comparing differences in the efficacy of daily vs. three times per week TMP-SMX administration for the prophylaxis of PCP.

Since low cost and self-administration are significant benefits, one would think that TMP-SMX prophylaxis would clearly be the preferred choice for PCP prophylaxis when compared to aerosol pentamidine. While TMP-SMX has demonstrated good efficacy, it does have several potential drawbacks worth noting:

1. The incidence of allergic reactions or rash, when TMP-SMX is taken over an extended period of time, reportedly approaches 20 percent. If an allergy to TMP-SMX develops during its prophylactic use, it might be eliminated as one of the available drugs for the treatment of an *acute* episode of PCP. Sometimes, a desensitization procedure can be carried out that eliminates an allergy to TMP-SMX, but this procedure does not always work.

2. One of the potential side effects of TMP-SMX is bone marrow suppression, which contributes to low red and white blood cell counts. AZT, the presence of a chronic illness and HIV itself can all cause mild to severe bone marrow suppression. Accordingly, the addition of a drug that adds to this effect may not be advantageous.

3. Our bodies maintain a large population of healthful bacteria to aid in normal processes, such as digestion, and to help

prevent the overgrowth of pathogenic (unhealthy) organisms. Long-term administration of antibiotics, such as TMP-SMX, alters the normal population of bacteria present in the body and this may pave the way for the occurrence of viral, fungal and other diseases that might otherwise not have occurred.

One recent study, performed at the Johns Hopkins University School of Medicine in Baltimore, may have unwittingly highlighted the above effects. 1,048 patients with a prior history of PCP and less than 250 T-helper cells were followed for approximately two years. Of the two groups, 17 percent developed PCP while taking Septra while 22 percent developed PCP while taking aerosol pentamidine. In spite of this small difference favoring Septra prophylaxis, a time dependent analysis of the data showed AP prophylaxis was associated with improved overall survival.

Although I currently have more patients taking TMP-SMX for PCP prophylaxis than AP, I am concerned about the above issues. Since my overall philosophy is to try and avoid the use of chronic systemic medications as long as possible, I will often recommend AP for prophylaxis as long as the T-helper cell number is above 100 cells/mm^3 and the patient can afford it. Once the T-helper cell number falls below 100 cells/mm^3, I feel more comfortable with the systemic presence of TMP-SMX.

Dapsone

Dapsone is another oral medication that has been recommended for PCP prophylaxis. There are several dosing regimens that are currently being used. One study reported on using a dosage of 25 mg four times daily in patients with under 250 T-helper cells. Over an average follow-up period of 9.4 months, two of these 173 patients were diagnosed with PCP. A second study published in the *Journal of AIDS* compared Dapsone 100 mg per day with TMP-SMX one double strength tablet per day. During 1,638 patient-months of observation, one episode of PCP developed in each group. However, side effects eventually necessitated the discontinuation of the drugs in a majority of patients in both groups. Cross-over from one drug to the other after the occurrence of a significant side effect was possible.

Dapsone does seem to have a lower incidence of allergic reactions than Septra. Even though it is a sulfa-type medication (a sulfonamide), if a person is allergic to TMP-SMX, they can often take dapsone without difficulty.

Dapsone, as well as TMP-SMX, can contribute to the occurrence of anemia, especially in patients who have a G6PD (Glucose-6-phosphate-dehydrogenase) deficiency. This is a genetic enzyme deficiency that occurs in less than 5 percent of the U.S. population. There is a lab test that can screen for this deficiency and I recommend that it be done for anyone who is considering long term dapsone use.

Dapsone is inexpensive, well tolerated, and does not have the wide range of bactericidal (antibiotic) activity that is inherent with TMP-SMX. This means that it does not alter your normal healthful bacteria quite as much. This could be a significant advantage when comparing it to other antibiotics.

Dapsone may also protect against other opportunistic infections, such as toxoplasmosis and MAI. These attributes make regimens containing dapsone especially attractive for PCP prophylaxis. I most frequently use dapsone in patients who are intolerant or allergic to TMP-SMX. The dosage I use is 100 mg three times per week for patients with greater than 100 T-helper cells/mm^3 and 100 mg daily for patients with below this number. In patients with less than 50 T-helper cells/mm^3, I often add an aerosol pentamidine treatment (300 mg) once every other month. I have had extremely good results with this regimen. See facing page for a summary of prophylaxis choices.

Toxoplasmosis Prophylaxis

When an HIV-positive individual has less than 100 T-helper cells, the incidence of opportunistic infections other than PCP begins to rise. Toxoplasmosis, a parasitic infection of the nervous system, is one opportunistic infection that occurs with a higher frequency below this T-helper cell number. Patients who are at this level should find out whether they have been exposed to toxoplasmosis by asking their physician to check their antibody level to this or-

PCP Prophylaxis Choices

Aerosol pentamadine

Pluses:
Several years of proven efficacy at a once monthly dosage of 300 mg.

Minuses:
Costly. Usually not administered by the patient.
May allow PCP to develop outside the lungs.
Not as effective as TMP-SMZ or Dapsone.

TMP-SMX

Pluses:
Inexpensive. Patient administered. Good efficacy. May also prophylax against Toxoplasmosis.

Minuses:
Twenty percent incidence of allergic reactions. Allergy may eliminate the ability to use in acute cases of PCP unless desensitization procedure is successful.
May contribute to lower red and white blood cell counts. Possibly distorts the body's natural balance of healthful bacteria.

Dapsone

Pluses:
Inexpensive. Patient administered. Good efficacy. May also prophylax against other opportunistic infections.

Minuses:
May contribute to anemia and peripheral neuropathy.

ganism. Several studies have been performed to gauge the prevalence of toxoplasmosis exposure in the gay population. They estimate that approximately 10 percent of gay and bisexual men have IgG antibodies to toxoplasmosis that were produced upon initial exposure to the organism. If this blood test is positive, and you have below 100 T-helper cells/mm^3, then prophylaxis against toxoplasmosis is warranted. If your antibody test comes back negative, you have probably not been exposed and there is less reason to take prophylaxis against this infection.

The *average* T-helper cell number at the time of toxoplasmosis diagnosis was reported in a study at the Seventh International Conference on AIDS (1990) to be between 50 and 60. Of patients with acute toxoplasmosis, 84 percent had T-helper cell counts less than 100.

The following drugs have been shown to have potential for prophylaxing against toxoplasmosis: TMP-SMX (Septra and Bactrim), dapsone, pyrimethamine, clarithromycin and azithromycin. The latter two drugs and dapsone are of particular interest because they have also shown activity against MAI infection. The dosages that are being tested include TMP-SMX, 1 double-strength tablet every other day; dapsone 100 mg 3x a week; pyrimethamine 25 mg 3x a week and clarithromycin 250 mg once daily.

Additional studies need to be completed before definitive recommendations can be made for prophylaxing against this infection. My current recommendation is that individuals with less than 50 T-helper cells/mm^3 take either TMP-SMX 1 double strength tablet or Dapsone 100 mg every day. Dapsone may also help prophylax against MAI as described below.

MAI (Mycobacterium Avium Intracellulare) Prophylaxis

MAI infection is caused by several different strains of Mycobacterium avium bacteria. Due to the presence of these multiple strains, MAI is often referred to as MAC, which stands for Mycobacterium avium complex. In its most aggressive form, MAI infection can cause high fevers, chronic anemia, malabsorption, weight loss and diarrhea. However, many people with AIDS have these organisms present in their bodies without experiencing any symptoms whatsoever. In autopsies, MAI organisms have been found in 50 to 70 percent of AIDS patients at the time of death. Many of these individuals were either asymptomatic or their infection was never identified.

MAI organisms are related to the organism that causes tuberculosis. The problem is that many single antibiotics are ineffective to adequately treat these infections. Tuberculosis is usually treated with a combination of three different antibiotics. MAI has been treated with anywhere from one to six antibiotics concurrently with varying results. Recently a drug from Europe, known as clarithromycin, has been used in the treatment of MAI with positive results. It is now available in the U.S. for the treatment of acute bronchitis and is used frequently as a first-line treatment for MAI (combined with clofazimine and others). A related medication, azithromycin, also appears to have significant anti-MAI activity.

Since clarithromycin and azithromycin have turned out to be relatively effective, well-tolerated treatments for active MAI, they may also provide effective prophylaxis for HIV-positive individuals at high risk for this infection.

In an abstract presented at the Seventh International Conference on AIDS (1990), 75 percent of the patients found to be culture-positive for MAI had less than 50 T-helper cells. There were no patients culture-positive for MAI with greater than 100 T-helper cells. Additionally, while only 18 percent of the patients tested had positive blood cultures for MAI, all of the patients with positive cultures were symptomatic. Therefore, patients at high risk for the presence of MAI are those with less than 50 T-helper cells and with symptoms such as fever, persistent anemia, weight loss and fatigue.

The following medications have been shown to have anti-MAI effects:

1. The antibiotics clarithromycin and azithromycin have been shown to achieve high concentrations in the body and

are active against both MAI and toxoplasmosis. There is currently an AIDS Clinical Trials Group study investigating the effectiveness of clarithromycin 1,000 mg twice daily versus placebo as primary prophylaxis against MAI. Many patients and physicians in the community have been experimenting with one 250 mg tablet of clarithromycin per day as MAI prophylaxis with beneficial results on an anecdotal basis. I advise my patients with less than 50 T-helper cells to take clarithromycin 500 mg 3 times per week, and I have not seen a new case of MAI amongst them in the eighteen months since beginning this regimen.

2. Clofazimine has been demonstrated to be effective in the experimental treatment of MAI infection and is currently being studied as a primary prophylaxis agent at a dose of 50 to 100 mg per day versus no treatment in 100 patients with AIDS. However, a study of this medication coordinated by the San Francisco County Consortium was recently called off because clofazamine appeared to show no benefit for preventing MAI infection when compared to a placebo.

3. Rifabutin has been shown to have both in vitro and in vivo activity against MAI. In one study, twenty-two patients were treated with rifabutin 300 to 900 mg per day and compared to 184 other AIDS patients in terms of survival and diagnosis of MAI infection. A trend towards prolonged, MAI-free survival was observed in the rifabutin-treated group after the drug was administered for greater than thirty days. This agent is currently being prospectively studied as a primary prophylactic medication by the Community Research Initiative at several centers across the United States. Preliminary results appear positive and Rifabutin may, in fact, become the first FDA approved drug for the prophylaxis of this infection.

4. Dapsone is also known to be active against MAI in laboratory studies. Since dapsone is also effective against PCP and toxoplasmosis, it may turn out to be an effective prophylaxis medication for the prevention of several opportunistic infections in patients with AIDS and low T-helper cell numbers.

It is currently my recommendation, based on my experience and the information now available, that individuals with T-helper cell counts less than fifty consider taking clarithromycin 500 mg 3 times per week for MAI prophylaxis. Since this medication is to be taken for the rest of an individual's lifetime, I recommend taking it 3 times per week instead of daily to allow the major organs of the body (the liver, kidneys and bone marrow) to rest and recover on the days they are not exposed to the medication. Additional studies are definitely necessary to document the efficacy of this and other long-term prophylaxis regimens.

Fungal Prophylaxis

Once an HIV-positive individual has less than 100 T-helper cells, the occurrence of fungal infections becomes increasingly likely. Fungi are one-celled organisms that are responsible for producing many different kinds of infections in people with AIDS. The decreased effectiveness of the cell-mediated arm of the immune system causes the immune system to be deficient in its ability to fight off fungal infections. The most common fungal infections found in people with AIDS are candidiasis (thrush), fungal infections of the skin and nails, cryptococcal meningitis and less commonly histoplasmosis, an infection of the lungs.

Although a definitive study has not proven the efficacy or safety of antifungal prophylaxis below a certain T-cell number, I generally, along with many of my colleagues in clinical practice, recommend fluconizole (Diflucan) 100 mg, taken 3 times per week, as safe and effective antifungal prophylaxis if the T-helper cell count falls below 50. This regimen has been well tolerated and appears to help reduce the incidence of fungal infections. Fluconizole is probably more effective than ketoconazole (Nizoral) and is less damaging to the liver. However, it is about three times as expensive. If cost is a problem, try Nizoral first. The comparable dosage of Nizoral is 200 mg, 3 times a week.

CMV (Cytomegalovirus) Prophylaxis

CMV infection is *the most common viral opportunistic infection seen in AIDS patients.* Once activated in an immune-compromised host, CMV is extremely aggressive and can cause fever, weight loss, chronic diarrhea, gastrointestinal ulcers and blindness. Almost 100 percent of gay and bisexual men with HIV infection test positive for exposure to CMV. The possibility of CMV's becoming active is much greater when the T-helper cell number is below 50 cells/mm^3.

Current options for prophylaxis against CMV reactivation are limited. There is an antibody test that can be obtained to document prior exposure to this virus; however, as mentioned above, almost 100 percent of gay and bisexual men will test positive. Some data are available suggesting that acyclovir, taken in extremely high doses, 800 mg four to five times daily, may be an effective pro-phylaxis. However, this high a dosage of acyclovir brings with it difficulties in both compliance and the possibility of side effects such as headaches, malaise, and crystallization of the drug in the renal tubules (similar to kidney stones).

Clinical trials are also under way for utilizing an oral form of DHPG, the I.V. medication currently used to treat acute CMV, as a prophylactic drug. There are a small number of other possi-bilities that are being tested in early experimental trials, including BW256U87, a drug that after digestion converts into a highly potent form of acyclovir.

The most important prophylactic measure to guard against CMV is to have an evaluation with an experienced ophthalmologist every 3 months when your T-helper cell count is less than 50 cells per mm^3. Prompt diagnosis and treatment of this infection can be both sight and life-prolonging. The time to catch CMV is *before* it affects your sight!

Immunizations

In HIV-positive individuals, vaccines play an important role in preventing common infections that can act as cofactors and stimulate additional HIV activity. Yearly immunizations for influenza and a one-time-only immunization with Pneumovax, a vaccine for the prevention of bacterial pneumonia, are currently recommended by the Centers for Disease Control and it's not a bad idea to add them to your treatment program. These vaccines are not known to interact negatively with antiviral medications and, in fact, have been demonstrated to show an enhanced effect when used in combination.

Hepatitis B vaccine has also been recommended for individuals who have never been exposed and therefore do not possess their own protective antibodies. However, if you are not routinely at risk of exposure through unsafe sexual practices or work in a medical or other health-care setting, I do not believe it is necessary that you receive this immunization.

TREATMENT OF SPECIFIC SYMPTOMS AND CONDITIONS

The treatment of specific symptoms should initially be discussed with your primary-care physician. However, in this section, I would like to present some of the beneficial knowledge that I have gained during my past five years of HIV-related experience.

As you read through the following list of symptoms and conditions, I hope that you will gain a clearer understanding of how to approach the most frequent "imbalances" which occur in HIV-positive individuals. The following symptoms and conditions are covered in this section:

- Candida

- Hairy Leukoplakia

- Fatigue

- Weight Loss

- Diarrhea

- Intestinal parasites
- Cryptosporidium
- Opportunistic Infections

Candida

Candida albicans is a fungus that is occasionally present in the mouth. It usually does not overgrow unless a person's immune system is weakened. When it overgrows, it is called thrush. Oral thrush is characterized by a persistent white coating on either the tongue or the back and sides of the mouth and throat. It may be accompanied by soreness and pain upon swallowing.

While many individuals may have a white coating on their tongue, it may or may not be due to thrush. The only way to know for sure is to send a swab of the affected area to the laboratory for examination. While other conditions can mimic a white film on the tongue, whitish, cottage-cheese-like blotches on the sides or back of the mouth are almost always due to thrush. There are two ways to treat thrush. The first is to prevent it with dietary measures and good oral hygiene. The second is with the use of antifungal drugs that are available by prescription. It has been my experience that most individuals following the Comprehensive Healing Program for HIV do not develop thrush. The reason is that their immune systems are strengthened by the use of nutritional supplements and a proper diet.

The most important aspects of this preventive program are the avoidance of sugar, alcohol, and dairy products. All three provide nutrients (simple sugars) for the thrush to feed upon. *If thrush is present when you begin this program,* I would advise very strict adherence to avoiding these three items in your diet, in addition to using one of the antifungal agents listed below.

In addition, good oral hygiene, including flossing, brushing, and rinsing your mouth twice a day, are strongly advised. The specific rinses that I recommend to my patients are Listerine and Peridex (available by prescription). These can be supplemented with herbal rinses and, occasionally, dilute hydrogen peroxide (one part peroxide to five parts warm water) for additional benefit. The above measures are usually sufficient to prevent the occurrence of thrush. If thrush does appear, there are several antifungal drugs that can be effectively used to treat it. My personal preference is Mycelex troches. Dissolve one in your mouth three to five times per day. An inexpensive alternative to this is Nystatin vaginal suppositories. Dissolve one in your mouth three times per day.

Other preparations are available in liquid form, such as nystatin swish and swallow. This solution contains 50 percent sugar. Unfortunately, the pharmaceutical industry has not yet realized that since yeast and fungi feed on simple sugars, avoiding these sugars might have a beneficial effect. As proof of this, the Miles Pharmaceutical Company continues to send me sugar-laced hard candies to be placed in my waiting room so that patients will be reminded of how easy it is to dissolve their Mycelex troches in their mouth. I haven't figured out whether they are just poorly informed or if they are actually trying to promote the growth of thrush in my patients. Needless to say, these hard candies never make it into my waiting room.

Finally, your physician may recommend that you take a systemic medication to treat persistent thrush. One choice is Nizoral (also known as ketoconizole). This medication is very effective but also carries with it the potential for systemic side effects such as allergic reactions and liver inflammation. A newer antifungal agent, fluconizole, is more effective and may cause fewer side effects.

To reiterate, the best treatment of this condition is its prevention. Utilize your overall program to make sure that thrush does not become a problem. If it does occur, follow the above recommendations to make it more manageable.

Hairy Leukoplakia

Hairy leukoplakia is a common condition that appears as a white thickening of the mucous membranes on one or both sides of the tongue. It is often asymptomatic; however, some patients complain of a "furry" feeling on their tongue or a bad taste in their mouth. It is easily recognizable upon oral inspection. Hairy leukoplakia was first identified in HIV-positive individuals in 1981. It is most probably an activation of a latent Epstein-Barr viral infection that has previously been dormant.

Once again, "the best offense is a strong defense." The prevention of this condition is a much more favored approach than treating it once it occurs. I have found that prevention is accomplished by a strong overall natural-therapies program supplemented, in most cases, by the use of an antiviral medication.

There are several topical treatments that are partially effective against hairy leukoplakia. These include daily applications of tincture of gentian violet (available from your pharmacy), daily application of .05 percent Retin-A lotion (available by prescription), and the use of twice daily Peridex rinses. It also seems that hairy leukoplakia is worse in the presence of a *Candida* infection, so the first step should include treatment and eradication of this infection with the use of antifungal lozenges.

Fatigue

If fatigue is present, is is very important to adhere to the recommendations listed below:

- Rest often.

- Avoid alcohol and caffeine.

- Practice relaxation exercises at least twice daily (yoga, relaxation tapes, meditation, etc.).

- Utilize the Your Healing Hour exercise (found in the Emotional Healing chapter).

- Make sure that you are taking adequate vitamin and herbal supplements.

- Consider including an antiviral medication as part of your treatment program.

- Rule out the presence of an active opportunistic infection (PCP, MAI, etc.).

The most important thing to understand about fatigue is that your body is attempting to communicate with you. It is trying to let you know that it needs additional rest. If you listen to its signals and make the necessary changes in the amount of energy you expend, you can achieve a better balance and feel better. If you ignore these signals and don't get enough rest, you are only setting the stage for minor symptoms to progress into major ones. Try instituting the recommendations listed above. If your fatigue is not due to an active opportunistic infection, you should notice improvement within a few weeks.

If improvement does not occur, your physician should perform a thorough work-up, including at least a physical exam, lab work, and a chest X-ray, to determine its cause. Treatment of the following conditions, if present, can help improve your fatigue:

- anemia

- sinusitis

- intestinal parasites

- pneumonia

- tuberculosis

- adrenal gland insufficiency

- opportunistic infections (PCP, MAI, CMV, etc.)

Weight Loss

It is important to understand that the recommendations contained within the Comprehensive Healing Program for HIV, including the Immune Enhancement Diet, have been extremely effective at preventing weight loss in my patients. However, if you are unexpectedly losing weight, it is important to make a few modifications in the Comprehensive Healing Program.

First, if your current weight is ten pounds or more below normal, suspend the sugar and dairy restrictions and begin increasing your caloric intake as much as possible. Weight loss has a momentum that is difficult to reverse. Gaining weight requires sufficient calories, protein, and ,rest and usually necessitates including high-calorie foods such as ice cream and milk shakes in your diet. The goal needs to be to increase the protein and caloric content of your diet as much as possible.

An oral medication that can be taken to stimulate your appetite and help you gain weight is called Megace. Megace is a hormone that is extremely well tolerated and effective. The initial dosage is 40 mg three times daily. It should be tried as soon as possible if unexpected weight loss occurs.

These recommendations are based on my experience with patients who have come to me symptomatic. Some have needed to go into the hospital because of their weight loss. Others have begun on intravenous nutrition. The factors that turned their declines around were complete bed rest and a suspension of most of the sugar and dairy restrictions previously mentioned. This means consuming the above stated foods as much as their appetites would allow. This is recommended only if weight loss is occurring and *diarrhea is not present.*

If diarrhea is present, weight loss becomes even more difficult to treat. First, the cause of the diarrhea must be identified and treated medically. Second, dietary modifications must be made. Refer to the following section on the treatment of diarrhea for the specific dietary and supplement recommendations to be included in your treatment program. After the diarrhea has resolved, you can include the aforementioned high-calorie foods (ice cream, dairy products, and desserts) in your diet to regain your weight. However, if diarrhea is present, these foods will be too rich and concentrated for your system to digest. Poorly digested food particles will only stimulate additional diarrhea and a vicious cycle will be set up. Therefore, treat your diarrhea first and then work on building your weight back up.

Third, complete bed rest is extremely important. Only complete bed rest will allow your body to conserve sufficient energy to rebalance the digestive system. Your digestive system must return to balance if you are going to improve your level of health.

If the above recommendations are not successful, you may

want to discuss total parenteral nutrition (known as TPN) with your physician. TPN provides nutrition intravenously so your digestive system can rest. Subsequently, when you slowly reintroduce solid foods, the diarrhea may not recur. It is an extreme interventional approach, and the decision to use it must be made on an individualized basis along with your physician.

There are several nutritional supplements that can also be included in your diet to further increase its protein and calorie intake. These include Bear Valley Meal Pack Bars (400 calories, 16 grams protein each), Gainer's Fuel by Twinlabs (531 calories, 21 grams protein per serving), and Ensure Plus (355 calories, 13 grams protein per serving). If the Gainer's Fuel and Ensure Plus are too rich for your taste, they can both be diluted with additional water to increase their palatability.

Diarrhea

About 50 percent of HIV-positive individuals have diarrhea at some point during the course of their condition. Diarrhea can decrease the absorption of nutrients and lower your energy level. It is therefore important that this symptom be addressed quickly to prevent it from having a weakening effect on your body.

The treatment of diarrhea in the HIV-positive individual can be both a simple and complex task. In all cases, its treatment can be optimized by adjusting your diet. The goal is to provide food that is simple and easy for your gastrointestinal system to digest. My dietary recommendations include the following:

1. Rest often.

2. Avoid milk, cheese, and yogurt.

3. Avoid fried foods, oils, and mayonnaise.

4. Increase high-fiber, complex carbohydrate foods such as oatmeal, barley, rice, pasta, potatoes, cracked wheat, and whole grain toast.

5. Increase salt- and potassium-containing foods, including bananas, fruit juices, whole grains, potatoes, and green leafy vegetables.

6. Keep your diet "dry." This means decreasing the amount of fats and oils that you consume. It does not mean to decrease your water consumption.

7. Make sure fluid intake keeps up with fluid loss. The best fluids to drink are herb teas such as chamomile and peppermint, plain water, and nutritious broths. Electrolyte-replacement drinks such as Gatorade and Ricelyte (an over-the-counter pediatric electrolyte-replacement formula available in pharmacies) are also beneficial.

The Benefits of Rest

If diarrhea is present, it signifies a weakness or imbalance in the gastrointestinal system. This can be the sole problem, or an intestinal infection may also be present. Large amounts of rest (at least two to three uninterrupted hours per day with your feet elevated) are necessary to help rebalance and restrengthen your system. This will allow the above dietary measures to work most effectively.

Nutritional Supplements for Diarrhea

The above dietary recommendations are the first step in the initial treatment of diarrhea. Sometimes they may be all that is required to completely eliminate your symptoms. If they are not sufficient, the next step is to add the following nutritional supplements to help further strengthen and balance your digestive system: 2 acidophilus capsules (Twinlab Allerdophilus works extremely well) and 4 oat bran tablets with each meal. Oat bran tablets are high in fiber and help to absorb excess fluid and bile acids, while acidophilus bacteria help neutralize pathogenic (unhealthful) organisms and bring the digestive process back to balance. I cannot tell you the number of cases of diarrhea (not caused by infection) that I have successfully treated by utilizing the above regimen of dietary adjustment plus nutritional supplements.

If diarrhea persists for more than a week while on the above regimen, it is important that you consult your physician to have

1. Routine stool tests for ova and parasites from a reputable laboratory experienced in their collection and evaluation are usually sufficient to diagnose most intestinal parasite conditions.
2. At least two samples, collected on separate days, must be obtained for an adequate test. Studies done in the past have shown that three samples bring the probability of diagnosing intestinal parasitic infections to approximately 90 percent. It is sometimes necessary to turn in an additional set of samples if the initial tests were negative and your symptoms persist.
3. Several medications can inhibit the detection of intestinal parasites. These include antimotility agents (Lomotil and Imodium) and antibiotics. These medications should be discontinued for at least several days before samples are collected. After collecting a stool sample and filling the transport vial, shake the vial vigorously to mix the sample with the transport medium. This ensures that the sample is well preserved before it gets to the laboratory.
4. A variety of parasites can inhabit the gastrointestinal systems of HIV-positive individuals. *All of them need to be treated.* It is necessary to completely eliminate their effects as cofactors in order to avoid the progression of HIV disease.

Treatment of Intestinal Parasites

Recommendations for the treatment of intestinal parasites can range from alternative therapies (such as garlic and herbs) to strong prescription medications. Some of these treatments can be ineffective and time-consuming (many herbal and alternative treatments) or effective but highly toxic (Flagyl). In my experience, utilizing a combination of natural therapies along with an antiparasitic drug that is not absorbed from the intestinal tract (Humatin), gives the best balance between efficacy and an absence of side effects.

The following is the treatment regimen I have used with enormous success to eliminate intestinal parasites. It is extremely effective against *Blastocystis hominus, Endolimax nana, Iodamoeba bütschlii, Entamoeba histolytica, and Entamoeba coli.*

	FREQUENCY	DURATION
Humatin	3 times a day	7 to 14 days
Two 250-mg capsules		
Psyllium seed husks		
2 teaspoons added to water to juice	3 times a day	7 to 14 days
Black walnut tincture		
2 dropperfuls added to water or juice	3 times a day	7 to 14 days

The above regimen should be taken as follows: 2 capsules of Humatin with a full glass of water or juice to which 2 teaspoons of psyllium seed husks and 2 dropperfuls of black walnut tincture have been added. This mixture should be taken three times per day on an empty stomach (either ½ hour before or 2 hours after meals).

The entire regimen needs to be taken for seven to fourteen days depending on the severity of the infection and how long it has been present. Two weeks after completion of the above regimen, a repeat set of stool samples should be collected to make sure that the intestinal system is completely free of parasites. The treatment regimen may be repeated again if necessary. Stronger antiparasitic medications, such as iodoquinol and Flagyl, can be used as second-line therapy if the above regimen fails to completely eradicate the infection. In contrast to Humatin, these medications may be associated with increased side effects.

If you continue to have repeated parasitic infections that initially respond to treatment but then recur, you may have to institute an ongoing parasite prophylaxis program such as the one I have outlined below. This will help keep your gastrointestinal tract healthy over an extended period of time.

Cryptosporidium Infection

Cryptosporidium is a protozoan that is commonly found in the environment. Although it is easily cleared from the gastrointestinal tracts of HIV-negative individuals, *Cryptosporidium* can become an aggressive, life-threatening infection in HIV-positive persons.

There is no officially approved drug for the treatment of cryptosporidiosis. In the past, many physicians recommended that their patients with cryptosporidiosis go home and make their final preparations. I have never felt that the treatment of this infection was hopeless and, in fact, have had several treatment successes with the following step-wise approach.

Parasite Prophylaxis Program

1. Fiber	Psyllium seed husks (Metamusil)	1 tsp 2 times a day
2. Acidophilus	Twinlab Allerdophilus capsules	2 caps 2 times a day
3. Herbs	*Rotate to a different herb every 10 days to prevent resistance and side effects.*	
	a) goldenseal root capsules	2 caps 2 times a day
	b) black walnut tincture	3 droppers 2 times a day
	c) activated charcoal	2 caps 2 times a day
4. Medications	Humatin 250 mg (if necessary)	1 cap 2 times a day

Treatment for Cryptosporidiosis

Step 1:   Obtain frequent bedrest.
Step 2:   Follow the dietary and nutritional supplement guidelines contained in the section on treating diarrhea (p. 173). Include oat bran and acidophilus supplements with meals as discussed on p. 174.

Step 3:   Begin taking Humatin (500 mg three times a
            day). Take the psyllium seed husks and black
            walnut tincture along with the Humatin. Since
            Humatin helps alleviate the symptoms of cryp-
            tosporidiosis (diarrhea, gas, bloating, and so
            forth) but does not actually kill the organism,
            you may need to take this regimen indefinitely
            as long as it is working. You may be able
            eventually to decrease this dosage. Remember,
            while taking any prescription medication, you
            should be supervised by your physician.

Step 4:   If diarrhea continues, add Questran, one
            packet two to three times daily, to the above
            treatment regimen. Questran is a bile-acid
            binder and, although it does not treat the
            cryptosporidiosis directly, it may help alleviate
            your symptoms.

Step 5:   If all of the above interventions are not effec-
            tive at significantly controlling your symptoms,
            I recommend beginning Sandostatin subcuta-
            neous injections at a dose of 250 micrograms
            two to three times per day. This dose may be
            increased as necessary.

Sandostatin is the commercial preparation of somatostatin, a naturally occurring hormone that diminishes the secretion of fluid into the intestines. The Sandoz company is currently working on an oral preparation of this hormone to avoid the necessity of daily injections.

The above stepwise approach has been extremely effective in diminishing, and often completely eliminating, the diarrhea, abdominal pain, cramping, weight loss, and other symptoms of *Cryptosporidium* infection. It is a perfect example of how both natural and standard therapies can be combined into a compre-hensive program that achieves a better result than either of the two alone (steps 1 and 2 are natural therapies; steps 3, 4, and 5 are standard medical therapies).

Opportunistic Infections

The treatment of opportunistic infections lies solely in the realm of standard medicine. While the main focus of this book has been prevention, if opportunistic infections do occur, it is best to submit to the advice and recommendations of your physician. During the treatment of an opportunistic infection, you may continue with your natural-therapies program (diet, vitamins, and so on). It usually will not interfere with your standard medical treatment.

Since a detailed description of the treatment of opportunistic infections is beyond the scope of this book, you may refer to other sources if you want to learn the details of these treatments for yourself. For a detailed explanation of the standard medical options for treating opportunistic infections, I recommend *The Medical Management of AIDS,* edited by Merle A. Sande, M.D., and Paul Volberding, M.D.

The bottom line regarding the treatment of opportunistic infections is this: Your doctor should be someone that you trust to advise you adequately if an opportunistic infection occurs. This is what they have been trained for and what they do best.

COFACTORS

There is currently speculation regarding the possibility that one or more cofactors are necessary to destroy the immune system in concert with the HIV infection. Several prominent scientific researchers, including Dr. Luc Montagnier, the codiscoverer of HIV, and Dr. Peter Duesberg, a University of California virologist, have postulated that the proposed mechanism of action of HIV does not demonstrate a clear explanation for the effects that it produces. Additional infections, ranging from syphilis to *Mycoplasma* species, have been suggested as possible cofactors that play a role in accelerating the progression of the immune system's degradation.

The mechanism of action of these cofactors, and how they

stimulate HIV, is the subject of much debate and speculation. One or several cofactors may directly stimulate HIV to become more aggressive and accelerate its destructive tendencies or facilitate its action in a way that it becomes more damaging to the immune system.

Total Symptom Elimination

To promote a dormant viral state and prevent the progression of HIV, it is extremely important that an individual eliminate as many cofactors as possible. These are the very agents that, if left untreated, will make it impossible for a dormant viral state to occur.

When I say total symptom elimination, I specifically mean the elimination of chronic sinusitis, chronic bronchitis, intestinal parasites, genital herpes, chronic indigestion, and diarrhea. Whether you use natural or standard therapies for the treatment of these symptoms, it is important that you completely eliminate them so that the immune system is not in a chronically activated state. Achieving this goal takes a high priority in the standard medical portion of my program. When it is achieved, the immune system is less activated (stressed), allowing it to devote more of its energies to other important functions.

It is important for an HIV-positive individual to be aware of recent research showing that continuing to participate in unprotected sex has been associated with a more rapid progression of HIV disease. It is postulated that continued unprotected sex may expose an individual to either additional sexually transmitted pathogenic cofactors (gonorrhea, syphilis, herpes, etc.) or allow *additional HIV viral particles* to enter the bloodstream and potentiate an already existing infection. It is important to consider this fact when two HIV-positive individuals in a committed relationship are deciding whether to have protected or unprotected sexual relations. When you consider the amount of effort that goes into developing a dormant relationship with the particular strain and quantity of HIV in your body, it does not make sense to open the door to additional and, perhaps more virulent, strains.

Hidden Cofactors: Stress, Poor Nutrition, and Emotional Distress

It is disturbing that, for the most part, only microbes are looked upon as potential cofactors in this condition. In my experience, other important "cofactors" which allow HIV to break down the immune system's barriers include stress, emotional disharmony, and poor nutrition. These cofactors need to receive the same attention that microbial infections do. I believe that the Comprehensive Healing Program for HIV adequately addresses these cofactors. That is one of the main reasons for its success.

When you address stress, emotional disharmony, and poor nutrition in your treatment program, you are attacking several contributing factors that when unaddressed allow HIV to remain active and progress. Eliminating these cofactors helps your immune system stay strong.

Another reason why the treatment of these cofactors may help to keep you healthy is illustrated by the following hypothesis: John Maddox, editor of the influential scientific journal *Nature*, postulated that HIV may in some way cause one subset of T-cells to attack another subset of T-cells. This is an autoimmune process. Eventually, as more and more T-cells are destroyed, the immune system burns itself out.

This contention is supported by the fact that HIV antibodies have been found to occur in mice that have never previously been exposed to HIV but do have lupus, an autoimmune disease. Additionally, there is evidence that the body's own antibody response, not the virus, may be responsible for causing an autoimmune reaction which leads to progression and ultimately AIDS.

If this hypothesis is true, it would justify the importance of an aggressive program of nutritional support for providing the raw materials necessary for the immune system to maintain its long-term health. Keeping your stress low would also help the body to reduce its wear and tear.

Research into these possibilities may eventually provide us with a new approach to the treatment of HIV that incorporates modifying this immune system imbalance with standard therapies.

Until that time, the Comprehensive Healing Program for HIV is perfectly suited for providing stability, strength, and the highest degree of health for an immune system which may be affected by a slowly advancing autoimmune process.

EXPERIMENTAL THERAPIES

The therapies selected for review in this section hold substantial promise for clearing investigational and regulatory hurdles and ultimately making it into general use. Timely and accurate information regarding their status and the status of other up-and-coming investigational agents can be obtained by subscribing to the following publications:

AIDS Treatment News
ATN Publications
P.O. Box 411256
San Francisco, CA 94141
(415) 222-0588

Treatment Issues
GMHC (Gay Men's Health Crisis)
Medical Information
129 W. 20th Street
New York, NY 10011
(212) 337-3695

BETA (Bulletin of Experimental Treatment for AIDS)
SF AIDS Foundation
P.O. Box 2189
Berkeley, CA 94702-0189
(800) 327-9893

D4T (Stavudine)

Background: D4T belongs to the nucleoside analog family of drugs, the same as AZT, ddI, and ddC. These medications terminate the DNA replication pathway of the virus before it is complete. D4T appears to increase T cells and decrease HIV replication. Bristol-Myers makes both D4T and ddI.

Recent studies: The largest studies to date have been performed by Dr. Lisa Dunkle. Combined data from six phase I and phase II trials totaling 264 patients throughout the U.S. were presented at the Harvard-Amsterdam AIDS conference in 1992. Improvements in T-4 counts of up to 50 percent or greater were seen in some patients and were sustained for a year. Other beneficial effects included declines in P-24 antigen levels, weight gain, and an enhanced sense of well-being. The doses that were tolerated best were 2 mg per kilogram of body weight per day.

Another study with 38 HIV-positive patients with less than 500 T-4 cells at entry showed that D4T reduced HIV levels in peripheral mononuclear cells and decreased acid-dissociated P-24 antigen levels at 2 mg per kg per day, but not at lower doses, after ten weeks of therapy.

An additional study showed that D4T had cognitive-enhancing effects similar to AZT in patients with HIV dementia. This finding suggests that D4T crosses the blood-brain barrier and is effective within the central nervous system.

Side effects: Peripheral neuropathy, elevated liver enzymes, headache, and nausea have all been seen at higher doses.

Current status: D4T was made available in October 1992 through its manufacturer, Bristol-Myers, in an expanded access program. In this program, any individual failing or intolerant to AZT and ddI should be able to obtain D4T free of charge through his or her physician, as long as peripheral neuropathy is not present.

Conclusion: D4T apparently will provide HIV-positive patients and their physicians another choice in standard nucleoside analog antivirals. This is especially good news for patients who have failed or are intolerant to AZT, ddI and ddC but who have not experienced peripheral neuropathy. Clinical studies will need to continue accumulating data before any statements can be made as to the relative potency of this medication when compared to the other drugs in its class.

Therapeutic Vaccines

Background: The goal of most vaccines is to prevent an individual from initially becoming infected with an infectious disease. The goal of HIV vaccine development is additionally geared to finding a vaccine that will enhance the immune response of an individual *who has already been infected* with HIV. Since HIV is a complex virus that mutates (changes its genetic code) rather readily, finding a vaccine that will produce effective and long-lasting antibody titers (levels) is a difficult task. Furthermore, vaccines are effective only in individuals who can mount an effective antibody response to a stimulus, thereby eliminating a large group of patients with advanced immune system destruction from benefiting from this form of treatment. However, for those individuals with immune systems still intact, HIV vaccines provide a hopeful means for maintaining an augmented immune response over a sustained period of time.

Recent studies: There are at least ten different HIV vaccines currently in clinical trials in the U.S. Most of the trials require that an HIV-positive individual have at least 400 T-helper cells to insure an adequate immune response to the vaccine's stimulus. At the VIII International Conference on AIDS held in Amsterdam (July 1992), Dr. Robert Redfield and his colleagues at the Walter Reed Army Hospital in Washington, D.C., reported on the use of a genetically engineered treatment vaccine from the MicroGeneSys Company in 30 HIV-positive men for almost three years. Their results suggested that injection with the gp160 vaccine boosts the immune system of individuals with HIV disease and between 400 and 700 T-helper cells. Of the vaccinated volunteers 83 percent displayed clear evidence of an increased anti-HIV response. Blood drawn from the 8 individuals receiving placebo vaccines showed no evidence of an increased anti-HIV immune response. The researchers have concluded that vaccine therapy with gp160 treatment vaccine induces an increased anti-HIV immune response in about 70 percent of treated individuals.

A team of researchers headed by Dr. Fred Valentine of New York University Medical Center also studied the safety and immune-enhancement potential of the gp160 vaccine from MicroGeneSys. This team studied 52 healthy HIV-positive volunteers with T-helper counts above 400. No adverse effects from the vaccine were reported other than slight skin irritation at the injection site. Shortly after receiving the gp160 treatment vaccine, all subjects experienced new and enhanced anti-HIV immune responses. Those receiving an alternate hepatitis vaccine did not develop these responses. Dr. Valentine said the next step in gp160 research will be to find out the lowest T-helper cell number above which patients still respond to the vaccine.

Side effects: There was initial fear that therapeutic HIV vaccines might stimulate increased HIV activity and thereby be detrimental to individuals who were HIV-positive. This has to date turned out to be untrue. Other than irritation at the injection site and rare elevation of liver enzymes, therapeutic HIV vaccines appear to be safe in individuals with greater than 400 T-helper cells.

Current status: Multiple clinical trials are currently enrolling participants. Widespread use and FDA approval for routine treatment in HIV disease are still probably several years away.

Conclusion: Therapeutic HIV vaccines appear to be safe and initially effective for individuals with greater than 400 T-helper cells. They are philosophically similar to natural therapies in the fact that they stimulate the body to produce a stronger immune response than it is presently mounting against HIV. I would strongly suggest combining vaccine therapy with the natural therapy recommendations of the Comprehensive Healing Program for HIV to provide the body with enhanced nutritional support during therapeutic vaccine therapy.

Mepron (Atovaquone)

Background info: Previously known as 566c80 Burroughs-Well-come's Mepron is a broad-spectrum antiprotozoal compound that has shown early signs of efficacy against *Pneumocystis,* toxoplasmosis, and *Cryptosporidium.* It is now in clinical trials for all three aforementioned infections and appears to be headed for timely approval for the treatment of mild to moderate PCP. It is an oral drug that must be taken with food (a high-fat meal is optimal) to be absorbed into the bloodstream.

Recent studies: A study conducted by Dr. Judith Falloon and coworkers at the National Institutes of Health was recently published in the *New England Journal of Medicine.* In this trial, 34 patients with mild to moderate PCP took three different doses of Mepron. All patients survived their pneumonia, and 79 percent were successfully treated with Mepron alone. Of the 34 patients, 5 did not respond, 2 developed a rash, and 2 a fever; 9 patients had rises in liver enzymes, but none had to stop therapy as a result of this side effect. Most of the participants were treated as outpatients. All of the doses seemed to be effective in treating PCP. The dose that was chosen for further testing was 750 mg taken three times daily with food.

A larger study that compares Mepron to TMP-SMX (also known as Bactrim or Septra) for PCP treatment is currently being conducted at thirty-nine sites throughout the United States, Canada, and Europe. Early analysis of the data suggests that patients treated with Mepron have nearly as good a response to therapy as patients treated with TMP-SMX. Of the patients treated with TMP-SMX, 25 percent had to discontinue therapy because of side effects, compared to only 10 percent with Mepron. However, it seems that more patients failed to respond to Mepron than failed to respond to TMP-SMX.

Animal studies show that Mepron is also effective at killing *Toxoplasma gondii,* the parasite responsible for an infection that can affect the nervous system of individuals with very low T-cell counts (T-4 count less than 100). Several small studies in humans have also had positive findings. Trials using Mepron to treat toxoplasmosis in patients with AIDS are currently ongoing at several centers throughout the U.S. If the results of these trials are positive, Mepron may be released in an expanded access program for the treatment of this infection.

Since Mepron is an oral drug, it may be able to be used as prophylaxis for both PCP and toxoplasmosis, in similar fashion to TMP-SMX. Studies are currently in development to test it in this fashion. The manufacturer is also working on a formulation that is less dependent on food intake for optimal absorption of the drug.

Side effects: Rash, headache, diarrhea, fever, elevated liver enzymes, and nausea are seen in 10 to 25 percent of patients taking the drug. For the most part, these effects have been mild and usually do not require cessation of therapy.

Current status: In September 1992, the FDA's Antiviral Advisory Committee recommended that Mepron be approved for the treatment of mild to moderate PCP. It will probably be available by prescription by the time you read this. Studies are still continuing to determine whether it is safe and effective for PCP prophylaxis, toxoplasmosis prophylaxis, and the treatment of *Cryptosporidium* infection.

Conclusion: Mepron appears to be an effective and relatively well-tolerated drug for the oral treatment of mild to moderate *Pneumocystis* pneumonia. It may also be effective for use in toxoplasmosis, cryptosporidiosis, and prophylaxis against PCP.

Protease and Tat Inhibitors

Background info: Protease inhibitors have a different target on HIV from other antiviral drugs. AZT, ddI, ddC and D4T are nucleoside analog medications that function by blocking HIV from copying its genetic information through the inhibition of the enzyme reverse transcriptase. Protease inhibitors block HIV's ability to replicate itself by inhibiting the protease enzyme. This enzyme is responsible for cleaving large viral sections, which when pieced together, form new copies of HIV.

Tat inhibitors aim at blocking the expression of a particular gene on the HIV genome, known as the tat (or transactivator) gene. This gene is responsible for "turning up the level" of HIV reproduction in infected cells.

Recent studies: The main problem in the development of protease inhibitors has been that the drugs appear to be poorly absorbed into the bloodstream following oral administration. Reporting at the Harvard-Amsterdam conference, Dr. Daniel Norbeck of Abbott Laboratories stated that an oral form of the medication, named A-80987, achieved good plasma levels in rats, dogs, and monkeys following oral administration. The drug also significantly inhibited HIV activity in the test tube. It entered phase I clinical trials in the fall of 1992. Unfortunately, Dr. Michael Otto of DuPont showed that HIV strains could become resistant to protease inhibitors after developing just a single mutation. This type of easy resistance development also sealed the fate of the much-touted TIBO (tetrahydroimidazobenzodiazepine) antivirals in 1992.

A phase I trial of tat inhibitors was also presented at the Harvard-Amsterdam conference. In this study, Dr. Paul Lietman from Johns Hopkins University reported on three groups of patients that received dosages of 60 mg, 200 mg, and 600 mg of the tat inhibitor drug, or a placebo. Accumulation of the drug over time was noticed at 600 mg, so this dosage level may eventually be dropped. Mild side effects were noted in 16 of 18 patients. The most common were headache, discoloration of the urine, and drowsiness.

Side effects: Protease inhibitors are reported to have minimal side effects. The side effects from tat inhibitors include headache, drowsiness, and discoloration of urine.

Current status: Several of the drug companies involved in researching these antiviral alternatives are earmarking large sums of money in the race to bring them to market. Phase I and II trials are currently being set up to test different formulations of these two classes of medications. Check the hospitals in your area or call 1-800-TRIALS-A for more information on how to participate in these studies.

Conclusion: Since these drugs work synergistically with AZT and other nucleoside analog medications, they may be able to be used in combination therapy. The goal would therefore be to suppress HIV activity at several different sites of its expression, enabling patients to have additional and potentially more effective options in suppressing HIV activity. Unfortunately, the development of these medications is running into difficulties that have also been encountered in the past with other potentially useful drugs: problems with absorption, resistance, and side effects, especially drowsiness with the tat inhibitors. These side effects might affect the quality of life of people who may need to take this drug for many years at a time. Hopefully these obstacles can be overcome in a timely fashion so that these promising drugs may achieve their potential.

CASE HISTORIES: EXAMPLES OF VIRAL DORMANCY

In this section you will become familiar with the personal stories of several of my "star players," patients who have learned to make the changes necessary to grow at a healthy and vibrant pace. These changes, by encouraging HIV to remain dormant, have enabled their immune systems to stay strong. Through these examples, I hope you can see the lifestyle adjustments that are necessary to stimulate your immune system, keep it healthy, and help keep you alive for a very long time!!

Patient 1

Carl and I first met in February 1988. He had originally tested HIV-positive in December of 1986 but believes that he was exposed much earlier. Carl was interested in reducing his stress and beginning a good nutritional program to help maintain his health. At the time, Carl was eating a diet that consisted of large amounts of red meat, fried foods, dairy products, processed sugars, and fat, all of which are unhealthful when consumed in large quantities.

After several visits, Carl returned to the macrobiotic-oriented diet that he had eaten in the early 1980s. This diet consisted of brown rice, whole grains, vegetables, and vegetable-based proteins such as beans, legumes, tofu, and tempeh.

When Carl and I originally began working together, his symptoms included intestinal gas, heartburn, excessive weight gain, and shoulder pain. All of these symptoms have now resolved. He used to drink alcohol every day, especially after work. Now he has quit entirely and regularly attends AA meetings. His most persistent negative health habit has been cigarette smoking, and after trying to quit several times, he has recently become successful.

Carl's most impressive achievement, to date, has come in the area of his work activities. He had previously been working in several stressful and unsatisfying job environments. After many job changes, he has now had a spiritual awakening. Carl has joined the Zen Buddhist Center in San Francisco and recently quit his job to move to the Tassajara Zen Center in central California for a six-month work-related sabbatical. He seems to be very happy with his decision, although he appears to have an understandable amount of apprehension due to such an unconventional change in his lifestyle.

Carl has had no HIV-related symptoms since an initial case of shingles in October of 1988. Carl participates in a monthly HIV support group and exercises with weights several times a week. His lab values are as follows:

DATE	T-4	T-8	RATIO	P-24	BETA-2
10/88	234	572	0.4	N/A*	N/A
1/89	353	1,004	0.3		
4/89	393	832	0.5		
7/89	374	833	0.4		
10/89	272	748	0.4		
1/90	375	735	0.5		
5/90	390	598	0.6		
8/90	392	682	0.6		
10/90	270	510	0.5		
1/91	468	918	0.5		
3/91	234	414	0.6		
7/91	520	920	0.6		
10/91	384	880	0.4		
2/92	352	816	0.4		

Medications: none.
Symptoms: none.
*Unavailable or not tested

Lab interpretation: In October 1988, Carl's T-4 number was 234. By February 1992, 3½ years later, his T-4 number had climbed to 352 and his ARC symptoms had entirely resolved. His helper/suppressor ratio is currently identical to what it was three years ago. Presently, Carl does not take any medications. In my opinion, his immune system is stronger because of the positive changes he has made in his diet and lifestyle.

Patient 2

John initially tested HIV-positive in June of 1988. When he first came to see me in July of 1990, John had already instituted a pretty impressive healing program. It included the use of vitamins, herbs, regular exercise, and some stress reduction techniques. His diet was fairly healthful, except that he often consumed foods with excessive amounts of processed sugar, especially when he was under a lot of stress.

What is most interesting about John's progress is that a few small but significant changes have really given his immune system a boost. These changes included decreasing his heavy intake of processed sugar, improving his stress reduction program with the addition of relaxation tapes, and eliminating his intestinal parasites (*Iodamoeba bütschlii* and *Endolimax nana*) utilizing the medication Humatin.

John has declined to take any antiviral medication. When one considers his remarkable progress to date, this decision appears to have been appropriate. His laboratory values are as follows:

DATE	T-4	T-8	RATIO	P-24	BETA-2
10/89	237	696	0.30	neg.	2.0
7/90	332	885	0.38	neg.	2.0
11/90	300	704	0.43	neg.	2.0
2/91	377	841	0.45	neg.	1.8
5/91	369	1,024	0.36	neg.	1.8
9/91	379	1,083	0.35	neg.	1.7
2/92	280	751	0.37	neg.	1.8
6/92	298	815	0.37	neg.	1.7

Medications: none.
Symptoms: none.

Lab interpretation: During the past three years, John's T-4 number has risen from 237 to 298. His helper/suppressor ratio has also improved during that time. The improved strenth of John's immune system appears to be directly linked to his aggressive natural-therapies and stress-reduction program.

Patient 3

Dennis is a forty-year-old gay man who originally tested HIV-positive in January of 1989. He believes that his initial exposure was back in the early 1980s. I began working with Dennis in November of 1989. At the time, Dennis complained of the following symptoms: tiredness, indigestion, irritability, frequent sinus infections, anxiety, depression, low T-helper cell count, and feelings of helplessness.

Dennis began his program by improving his diet. He completely eliminated all soft drinks, hard liquor, processed sugar, and other highly processed foods. He began eating breakfast every day, including lots of fresh fruit and vegetables in his diet, and drinking pure water and herb teas. Additionally, he decreased his dairy intake to no greater than 5 percent of his overall diet. All of these changes were made with the agreement that after a one-month trial, if he were not feeling significantly better, he could go back to eating whatever he wanted. One month later, Dennis returned for his follow-up visit stating, "My digestion has improved tremendously. I don't even miss coffee or sugar." He also said his new diet was not as hard to follow as he originally had thought it would be.

Next, we adjusted Dennis's vitamin and herb program by placing him on the Comprehensive Healing Program regimen. We increased his exercise to three times per week and had him begin listening to daily stress-reduction tapes. In April of 1990, Dennis began taking AZT 300 mg per day because of a positive P-24 antigen test. He continued to experience a decrease in his initial symptoms, including diminished digestive complaints, and an increase in his energy level as well as in emotional stability. Dennis also continued his regular emotional support group meetings and acupuncture treatments. Over the next year Dennis's symptoms completely resolved except for occasional sinus congestion. His T-helper cell number continued to climb.

When Dennis first came to see me, his diagnosis was ARC because of his chronic diarrhea, indigestion, fatigue, and low T-helper cell count. Two years later, he is almost completely asymptomatic. His lab tests are as follows:

DATE	T-4	T-8	RATIO	P-24	BETA-2
12/89	255	919	0.3	N/A	N/A
03/90	288	847	0.3	16	2.4
05/90	310	1,179	0.3	neg.	2.6
08/90	376	1,129	0.3	6	2.3
12/90	365	1,197	0.3	6	2.4
03/91	364	1,213	0.3	7	2.8
05/91	296	1,184	0.3	12	2.5
08/91	249	1,048	0.2	7	2.7
02/92	265	1,057	0.2	neg.	2.5

Medications: AZT 3 100 mg tabs per day (began 3/90), ddC 6 0.375 mg tabs per day (began 8/91).
Symptoms: occasional sinus congestion.

Lab interpretation: Dennis is a perfect example of a person who has made effective positive lifestyle changes as part of his healing program. Dennis's current program is very well-balanced, including a healthy diet, nutritional supplements, emotional support, and standard medications. It has been impressive to watch most of Dennis's chronic symptoms disappear as his program has been instituted. His T-4 counts are stable, his P-24 antigen level has become negative, and most importantly, he feels extremely well.

Patient 4

Bob was twenty-five when he initially tested HIV-positive in 1987. One year earlier, he had tested HIV-negative. At his first visit, he appeared extremely healthy and had no symptoms. He had already instituted a strong natural-therapies program including a healthful diet, vitamin and herb supplements, and regular exercise. Bob had quit smoking six months prior to our first visit and was now meditating regularly.

I was very glad to begin working with Bob because he is an example of a patient who I feel can do extremely well for a very long period of time. He is young, healthy, and highly motivated, and he began practicing the Comprehensive Healing Program for HIV very early in the course of his condition. My belief continues to be that if the Comprehensive Healing Program for HIV is begun early, there is *no reason to expect* an inevitable breakdown in the strength of the immune system.

Bob's first three visits were spent orienting him to the intricacies of the program. After that, I felt that he was well on his way physically, emotionally, and spiritually and would do well in the coming months. He has not needed to use any medications and has remained totally asymptomatic during the past several years. The following are his laboratory values:

DATE	T-4	T-8	RATIO	P-24	BETA-2
2/89	629	1,390	0.50	neg.	2.8
7/89	914	2,035	0.45	neg.	2.9
8/90	629	923	0.68	neg.	2.4
3/91	818	1,140	0.72	neg.	2.2
9/91	815	1,006	0.81	neg.	2.0
4/92	799	1,247	0.64	neg.	2.1
10/92	751	1,132	0.66	neg.	2.0

Medications: none.
Symptoms: none.

Lab interpretation: Bob's last values clearly indicate a strengthening of his immune system during the past two years. His T-helper cell number has increased by more than 100, his helper/suppressor ratio has improved, his P-24 antigen remains negative, and his beta-2 microglobulin has declined. Although Bob's healing program has been successful to date, it is important to realize that healing is a dynamic process that requires constant work. Bob will need to stay focused and committed to a process of continual growth for his immune system to remain healthy and strong.

Patient 5

Jim was thirty-four when he tested HIV-positive in 1988. He had been extremely healthy previously except for a mild case of hepatitis in 1978. Jim was very anxious about his health situation, so he set out to construct an aggressive healing program utilizing all of his knowledge and resources. His program included a natural-foods diet, the use of vitamin and nutritional supplements, regular exercise, and the rigorous practice of meditation, yoga, affirmation tapes, and Buddhist chanting.

This program was very difficult for Jim to maintain along with his regular job as a teacher of English. Things began to get fairly stressful as Jim realized that there were not enough hours in the day to do both. He was becoming increasingly uptight and tense about the difficulties of his situation.

During our initial discussions, we focused on the "rigidity" of his program. We agreed that he needed to have a more healthful and flexible approach to the situation, including more time spent relaxing and enjoying his life. It seemed that if he could just follow his heart's desires when it came to choosing the activities of the day and not be so hard on himself for not doing everything he "should," he might achieve a more balanced healing program.

Jim eventually retired from his job as an English teacher and now teaches yoga. He is much happier and healthier. Additionally, he has weekly sessions with a therapist, gets regular acupuncture treatments, and attends retreats out of the city as often as possible. You might think that Jim is independently wealthy, but he isn't. It is just that he has adjusted his priorities more toward his spiritual and health-care needs. Admittedly this approach is not for everybody, but it has worked for Jim.

Medically, Jim continues to remain asymptomatic and, in spite of a persistently positive P-24 antigen test, has maintained a stable T-helper cell number. Several times I have offered antiviral therapy to Jim to help strengthen his overall program, but he has refused. Instead, he prefers to focus all of his energies on his natural, spiritually oriented healing program which, as long as it continues to work, eliminates any disagreement on my part.

The following are Jim's lab values during the past four years:

DATE	T-4	T-8	RATIO	P-24	BETA-2
7/88	330	N/A	N/A	N/A	N/A
11/88	325	1,297	0.3	132	3.3
3/89	441	1,756	0.3	neg.	2.9
9/89	300	1,462	0.2	neg.	3.3
2/90	128	664	0.2	29	3.8
4/90	366	1,668	0.3	41	3.6
8/90	405	1,787	0.2	51	4.1
2/91	485	1,998	0.2	47	4.0
9/91	441	1,896	0.2	45	4.2
4/92	365	1,848	0.2	224	4.1
6/92	396	1,681	0.2	110	3.8

Medications: none.
Symptoms: none.

Lab interpretation: As I mentioned above, Jim's healing program is particularly strong when it comes to the natural, emotional, and spiritual elements. He has refused my suggestion to add antiviral therapy (because of his persistently positive P-24 level) and continues to prove that it is unnecessary for him based on his stable T-helper cell number and lack of symptoms. The T-cell test from February 1990, when his number dropped to 128, is probably an erroneous value. As long as Jim continues to follow his strong natural-therapies and emotional-healing program, I have no reason to believe that he cannot maintain this balanced state indefinitely.

Patient 6

Jake has always been a very interesting and challenging patient. When he initially came to see me, Jake was forty pounds overweight and extremely stressed and took medication for high blood pressure. He did not exercise, ate an unhealthful diet, and was holding in a lot of emotional pain. His initial motivation for coming to see me was to assist him with reducing his stress.

I have now seen Jake in therapy a total of sixty times during the past three years (average two times per month). Since our sessions began, Jake's high blood pressure has completely resolved. He has lost thirty pounds, and he exercises vigorously at a gym several times a week, assisted by a trainer. Much of Jake's anxiety regarding his HIV status has also been worked through. His HIV positivity is no longer a big secret that he is ashamed of.

To further reduce the stress in his life, Jake has retired from the corporate world and is now devoting his time and efforts to maximizing his healing program. As you can see from his lab tests, and from the fact that he has remained healthy over the last three years, Jake has proven the ability to strengthen his immune system with the Comprehensive Healing Program for HIV. The following are Jake's laboratory values:

DATE	T-4	T-8	RATIO	P-24	BETA-2
7/89	146	810	0.20	neg.	5.9
8/89	264	970	0.30	neg.	5.8
6/90	262	995	0.26	neg.	5.4
11/90	385	1,662	0.23	neg.	6.4
3/91	340	1,676	0.20	neg.	5.7
7/91	269	1,382	0.19	neg.	5.7
9/91	283	1,378	0.21	neg.	6.5
11/91	374	1,377	0.27	neg.	5.5

Medications: AZT 300 mg per day (since July 1989); fluconazole 100 mg three times per week; ddC three times per day (added in October 1991).
Symptoms: none.

Lab interpretation: Jake's T-4 count has improved by 150 percent since he began the program more than two years ago. His helper/suppressor ratio has also improved during this time. Most importantly, Jake feels better now than he has in a very long time. His program represents an excellent balance of natural and standard medical therapies.

Patient 7

Alan is a fifty-eight-year-old business executive who tested HIV-positive in 1986. Since that time, he has been very active in HIV emotional support groups that focus their attention on positive attitude and wellness. He occasionally attends a health-promoting weekend seminar and is very focused on continuing his growth and healing on every level.

When I first saw Alan in 1987, his diet was excellent, and he was following an extensive vitamin and nutritional-supplement program. He now meditates at least once a day for twenty minutes and is convinced that his emotional and spiritual focus has been extremely beneficial in maintaining his good health. Several specific techniques, including positive affirmations and daily readings from *A Course in Miracles* (a book devoted to spiritual growth), are responsible for his feeling less fearful and anxious. It is noteworthy that Alan and his lover have been together for thirty years.

Alan and I meet for quarterly follow-up visits that are often geared to helping him stay focused on his healing program. The following are Alan's lab tests from the past five years:

DATE	T-4	T-8	RATIO	P-24	BETA-2
5/87	621	1,373	0.45	N/A	N/A
3/88	640	1,320	0.50	N/A	N/A
8/88	660	1,220	0.50	N/A	N/A
5/89	700	1,150	0.60	neg.	2.4
8/89	550	1,120	0.50	neg.	2.7
11/89	590	910	0.65	neg.	2.6
5/90	650	1,320	0.50	neg.	2.5
8/90	840	1,850	0.45	neg.	2.7

1/91	617	2,214	0.30	neg.	2.4
5/91	580	1,340	0.40	neg.	2.5
9/91	620	1,250	0.49	neg.	2.2
12/91	900	1,800	0.50	neg.	2.1
3/92	710	1,510	0.47	neg.	2.4

Medications: none.
Symptoms: none.

Lab interpretation: Alan's case provides a perfect example of a dormant viral state. These laboratory values reflect an immune system that has remained stable during the past five years. The T-helper cell number is currently almost identical to what it was five years ago. The helper/suppressor ratio has also improved slightly, and his other parameters also continue to show stability. Alan's constant focus on his healing program has contributed tremendously to this stable state. He is always looking for new and creative ways to help his mind stimulate and strengthen his immune system. Alan has not needed any regular medications during this time.

Patient 8

Charles originally tested HIV-positive in 1986. He came to see me for his initial visit in 1988. At the time, he was trying to improve his diet and keep his stress low.

A central aspect of Charles's program has been relieving his feelings of emotional stagnation. He has always been a quiet individual who was not very open with his feelings. Everything had to be thoroughly thought through before he acted. Charles also felt that his life was becoming tedious and somewhat boring.

After several months of working with him, I recommended that he seek out more invigorating and stimulating activities that would give him pleasure; in other words, that he have more fun. I encouraged him to use the "positive affirmations" technique to break through some of the blockages that prevented him from enjoying himself. These suggestions and techniques have been very helpful to Charles. He now feels more worthy of receiving pleasure in his life.

On a medical note, Charles routinely tests positive for intestinal parasites. On two occasions he was treated, tested negative shortly afterwards, and once again tested positive several months later. I feel it is very important to *completely eradicate* intestinal parasites. They are cofactors that stimulate the HIV condition. I recommend checking for them frequently (at least once a year) and treating aggressively whenever their presence is detected. It is also important to understand how easy it is to be exposed to parasites, even while following routinely prescribed safe sex guidelines. Parasites can be contracted *much* more easily than HIV when one is exposed to infected bodily secretions.

Otherwise, Charles's health has remained extremely good. He follows the Comprehensive Healing Program for HIV faithfully, and the majority of our work has been focused on his emotional growth. The following are his laboratory values:

DATE	T-4	T-8	RATIO	P-24	BETA-2
9/88	378	577	0.60	N/A	N/A
1/89	748	2,020	0.40	N/A	N/A
8/89	464	793	0.60	neg.	2.1
12/89	730	1,266	0.60	neg.	2.3
3/90	426	767	0.60	neg.	2.4
6/90	434	813	0.50	neg.	2.0
9/90	517	931	0.56	neg.	2.0
1/91	581	871	0.67	neg.	1.9
4/91	528	989	0.53	neg.	2.4
9/91	454	952	0.48	neg.	2.0
12/91	462	781	0.59	neg.	2.2
3/92	514	962	0.53	neg.	2.3
10/92	590	1,386	0.43	neg.	2.2

Medications: none.
Symptoms: none.

Lab interpretation: Charles's case provides another example of a dormant viral state. His T-4 number is now higher than it was four years ago without the use of drugs. This case demonstrates the potential for the T-4 number to fluctuate widely, so it is important not to make any important decisions based on only one test. A more intelligent course of action is to observe the parameter for a pattern or trend. If there appears to be only an up-and-down fluctuation in the numbers, aggressive action with medications may not be necessary or warranted. Charles continues to remain entirely asymptomatic.

Patient 9

Ed is forty years old and has worked as an executive consultant for several nonprofit organizations. Although Ed tested HIV-positive in 1987, he believes that he was originally exposed in 1983. By the time we first met, Ed had constructed a healing program that included regular exercise, a healthy diet, and a regular program of stress reduction. He began the Comprehensive Healing Program for HIV in the summer of 1988. In the 3½ years since, he has remained in excellent health and does not exhibit any HIV-related symptoms. As his lab tests demonstrate, his T-helper cell number is higher now than when he first began the program.

DATE	T-4	T-8	RATIO	P-24	BETA-2
11/88	863	772	1.10	N/A	N/A
4/89	1,037	1,197	0.90		
8/89	1,050	950	1.11		
10/89	936	960	1.00		
1/90	1,386	1,221	1.10		
4/90	690	600	1.30		
8/90	966	943	1.00		
11/90	680	731	0.90		
1/91	630	616	1.00		
4/91	1,000	1,175	0.90		
8/91	912	1,272	0.70		
1/92	1,036	1,288	0.80		
7/92	925	1,100	0.80		

Symptoms: none.
Medication: none.

Lab interpretation: Ed's T-4 number has fluctuated widely. Between January and April 1990, the T-4 number dropped from 1,386 to 690. To the unskilled eye, this may appear to be a dramatic decline. However, if you also look at the T-8 number and the helper/suppressor ratio, you will see that both the T-4 and T-8 numbers declined to a similar extent. The ratio of the two was also higher in April than in January. Interpreting all of these numbers collectively helps you see that there was no cause for alarm, and, subsequently, the T-4 number went back up to 966. This patient's values highlight the need to identify the normal range of T-cell numbers that indicates stability for you. With this patient, I would say that anywhere between 600 and 1,000 is a safe and stable range for his T-4 number. If more than one lab test showed a decline below 600 T-4 cells, I would recommend treating in an aggressive fashion, either with a major lifestyle change or the addition of an antiviral medication.

I could go on and on. There are many more patients in my practice who have achieved viral dormancy by aggressively practicing the Comprehensive Healing Program for HIV. By working with the techniques I have described, you too can construct an individualized healing program that adds many productive and high-quality years to your life. Don't give in to the negative programming of those that say, "There is nothing you can do." Make positive healing changes in your life and start proving them wrong!

APPENDIX

COMPREHENSIVE HEALING PROGRAM FOR HIV-RESEARCH STUDY

Summary: The Comprehensive Healing Program for HIV research study was designed to determine whether a standardized program of natural therapies, when combined with appropriate standard medical care, would have a measurable influence on the course of HIV disease when compared to other groups treated with standard medical therapies alone.

All ten participants began this study in 1988 with a diagnosis of asymptomatic HIV-positive. They received a one-month orientation to the program and were then seen at three-month intervals for laboratory evaluation and routine physical examination.

We compared our data to the data of two other groups. The first was a similar group of asymptomatic HIV-positive men participating in a different study that was purely observational in nature. An assumption was made that the participants of this group were following the community standard of care. The second group comprised asymptomatic HIV-positive historical controls taken from the data base of the San Francisco Men's Health Study.

After a period of thirty months, the mean T-helper cell count of our study group declined by 4 percent (406 to 391). The mean red and white blood cell counts remained stable at 96 and 105 percent of baseline, respectively. The mean T-suppressor cell number rose by 27 percent. There was no mortality. There was only one opportunistic infection in the study group (PCP). This occurred at month twenty-eight of thirty in a participant who was not on PCP prophylaxis despite a T-helper cell count of 138 cells per mm³ at the start of the study. There were no other significant symptoms, serious infections, or disease progression in the other nine participants during the study period. In contrast, there was an 18 percent decline in the T-helper cell number of comparison group #1 and a 51 percent decline in the T-helper cell number of comparison group #2 during a similar period of time. Additionally, comparison group #1 had a mortality rate of 17 percent. The mortality rate of comparison group 2 was not reported.

Background

One of the medical dilemmas emerging from the current AIDS crisis is the advisability of treating asymptomatic HIV-positive individuals early in the course of their disease with potentially toxic therapies in order to beneficially influence the progression of their infection. Positive intervention in areas other than drug therapy might greatly benefit this patient population.

Although difficult to quantify, several lifestyle factors are known to negatively affect the functioning of the immune system. Poor nutrition and vitamin deficiencies can limit the immune system's reactivity and responsiveness to infections.[1,2] Stress, through a variety of mechanisms, alters the absolute number of T-helper cells and decreases the helper/suppressor ratio.[3,4,5] Presumably, treatment programs which are nontoxic and directed toward a reduction in stress and the provision of adequate nutrition could be beneficial to individuals who are chronically infected with HIV.

Finally, other healthful lifestyle practices such as moderate exercise and the elimination of negative health habits (such as smoking, alcohol, and recreational drug abuse) could be part of a comprehensive early intervention program whose goal it is to provide a means for HIV-positive individuals to optimize their general health and potentially decrease the speed of progression to symptomatic HIV infection, ARC, and AIDS.

This pilot study was designed to determine if a standardized program of early intervention with nonpharmacologic therapies, in addition to appropriate standard medical care, could reduce the progression of HIV disease in asymptomatic HIV-positive gay males, when compared to the course of two natural history comparison groups.

Methods

Ten asymptomatic HIV-positive individuals with varying T-4 counts were enrolled after answering an advertisement in the local San Francisco press. Each agreed to modify his diet and lifestyle as per the study protocol and to return at three-month intervals for follow-up laboratory and physical examinations. Laboratory parameters that were followed included CBC with differential, platelet count, T-4 and T-8 absolute numbers, and the helper/suppressor ratio. These parameters were monitored quarterly for the thirty-month study period. All laboratory analyses were performed at the University of California San Francisco Department of Laboratory Medicine. To eliminate the effects of diurnal variation in T-cell numbers, all blood draws were scheduled at the same time of day for each participant.

At the initial interview, participants were asked questions about their past medical history, present symptoms, and current lifestyle behavior. A five-day diet diary was also reviewed at the time of enrollment.

The participants were then asked to return on a weekly basis for one month to complete their nutritional counseling and orientation to the program. They subsequently returned on a quarterly basis for the remainder of the study period, at which time laboratory tests, a history, and a physical examination were performed.

The Study Protocol

All of the participants agreed to follow the program outlined below:

1. To consume a diet of adequate protein and calories consisting primarily of whole grains, fruits, vegetables, fish, poul-

try, eggs, seeds, nuts, herbs, and spices that are preferably naturally grown, locally harvested, and in season.

2. To take the following vitamins and nutritional supplements (provided at no cost): KAL Multi-Fours, 2 tabs twice daily; Twinlab Vitamin C 1000 mg, 2 caps twice daily; Twinlab Vitamin E 400 units, 1 cap twice daily; Twinlab beta-carotene 25,000 units, 1 cap daily; Twinlab Acidophilus, 1 cap twice daily; and RESIST (an astragalus-based herbal supplement containing several commonly prescribed oriental herbs), 4 caps three times a day.

3. To exercise on a regular basis no less than three times per week. Recommended exercise activities include walking, jogging, swimming, and weightlifting.

4. To refrain from the use of cigarettes, marijuana, alcohol, and other recreational drugs during the study period.

5. To listen to a fifteen-minute stress reduction tape twice daily.

6. To meet in a professionally facilitated emotional support group once monthly.

7. To continue the use of standard medical therapies (AZT, Septra, aerosol pentamidine, and so on) as prescribed by their primary care physician.

Results

Study Group Results

At baseline, the ten-member study group included five participants with T-4 numbers above 300 and five participants with T-4 numbers below 300. At the conclusion of the study thirty months later, this distribution was identical.

Additionally, at the thirty-month point of the study, the mean T-4 number of the study group was 96 percent of baseline (fig. 1). The hematocrit was also 96 percent of baseline (fig. 2). The mean white blood cell count of the study group rose by 5 percent and the T-8 count rose by 28 percent (fig. 3 and 4). Overall survival was 100 percent (fig. 5).

Two of the study participants began AZT therapy during the study period. Both took AZT as a result of T-helper cell declines that occurred while following the study protocol. The results of their T-helper cell values before and at the end of the study period are summarized in table 1.

Eight of the participants reported feeling better at the end of the study than before it began, a remarkable statement after thirty months of documented HIV positivity. There was one study participant who experienced disease progression. This occurred in an individual who began the study with 138 T-4 cells but who was not begun on PCP prophylaxis at that time. This participant had a prolonged episode of PCP at month 28 of 30 of the study but recovered after treatment with standard therapy.

The remaining nine participants experienced no incidence of significant symptoms, serious infections, or disease progression during the entire thirty months. There was no occurrence of fatigue, thrush, hairy leukoplakia, lymphadenopathy, diarrhea, dementia, or weight loss.

Comparison Groups

The baseline mean T-helper cell counts for the study group and two comparison groups were as follows: study group: 408 cells per mm³, comparison group #1: 476 cells per mm³, and comparison group #2: 698 cells per mm³.

Comparison group #1 was comprised of asymptomatic HIV-positive gay males who were being followed at the same laboratory during an identical period of time and who had the same medical tests performed as the study group. These individuals were not exposed to the study protocol in any way. It is assumed that they provide an accurate representation of the community standard of care during this time.

During our study period, comparison group #1 experienced a 17 percent mortality rate (3 of 18). When the last documented T-helper cell value of this group's deceased or lost to follow-up participants was carried through to the thirty month observation point, the group's mean T-helper cell number declined by 18 percent.

Data for a second comparison group (comparison group #2) was taken from the published observations of the San Francisco Men's Health Study.[6] This group consisted of 386 homosexual/ bisexual HIV-positive males. They were examined and tested at six-month intervals between 1984 and 1987 and are assumed to have followed the community standard of care at that time.

The mean T-helper cell number of comparison group #2 declined 49 percent during a comparable thirty-month period (an average loss of 84 cells per mm[3] per year). This compared with an observed decline in the T-helper cell number of our study group of only 4 percent. The T-4 declines of the study group and the two comparison groups are illustrated in Figure 6.

Discussion

It has previously been documented on numerous occasions that micronutrient deficiencies and gross malnutrition have adverse effects on immunologic functioning.[7,8] Studies of individuals with protein-calorie malnutrition and other nutrient deficiencies have shown a clear depression of cellular immunity including abnormal T-cell and macrophage function.[9] Based on extensive research, recommendations have been made by both the Task Force on Nutritional Support in AIDS and the American Dietetic Association to begin nutritional counseling as early as an HIV(+) diagnosis. This is rarely done in most community settings.[10,11]

It has been our experience that early and continued intervention with aggressive nutritional counseling needs to be the cornerstone of an integrated management plan for HIV disease. Ensuring optimal nutritional status can usually be counted upon to improve a patient's quality of life and might also prevent or diminish impairment of the immune system over time.[12] Identifying patients at risk for protein deficiency in the face of a chronic infection can help eliminate an especially serious and easily correctable cause of immunosuppresion.[13]

Additionally, there has been a tremendous amount of recent

research on the potential of various vitamin and mineral supplements to have a protective effect on the immune system. Vitamins C, B_6, E, beta-carotene, and the minerals zinc and selenium have all shown promise as modulators of immune system function.[14]

Although there has been a great deal of controversy on the merits of prescribing vitamin C in dosages that exceed the RDA recommendation of 60 mg per day, several studies have found that supplementary doses of 500 to 1,000 mg per day of this vitamin significantly increase blood levels of IgA, IgM, and C3. Vitamin C has also been shown to enhance the proliferative response of T lymphocytes in vitro,[15] and the tuberculin skin sensitivity of elderly volunteers is enhanced in vivo by vitamin C administration when compared to controls receiving placebo.[16] Harakeh, Jariwalla, and Pauling have shown that vitamin C, in high doses, demonstrates in vitro antiretroviral activity, including inhibition of P-24 antigen formation, equal to that of AZT.[17]

Medicinal herbs may be able to help asymptomatic HIV-positive individuals maintain strong immune function over time.[18] Interest of the Western medical community in the immunomodulatory effects of Oriental herbs, including astragalus and ligustrum, dates back to a landmark article published in the *Chinese Medical Journal* in 1981. This article documented greatly increased survival rates and a diminution of symptoms in cancer patients treated with a combination of standard medical therapies and Oriental herbs.[19]

Other studies by Chu and associates at the M.D. Anderson Cancer and Tumor Institute in Houston, Texas, have shown that purified fractions of astragalus root possess potent immune-restorative activity both in the test tube and in rats.[20] Dr. Chu and his coworkers found that by incubating astragalus root extract and white blood cells along with interleukin-2, a naturally produced immune system mediator, they produced a tenfold increase in the white blood cell's cytotoxic effect on tumor cells.

Dr. Chu's studies have also shown that a partially purified fraction of astragalus root when injected into rats who had previously been treated with high doses of cyclophosphamide (an immunosuppressant), was able to reverse this immunosuppression as manifested by the return of the rat's ability to reject xenografts.[21] Dr. Chu has suggested that these partially purified fractions of astragalus root be tested in phase I trials in patients suffering from diseases that produce immunodeficiency states such as that found in AIDS.

In addition to the above 'nutritional interventions, a regularly practiced exercise and stress management program has been shown to improve the functioning of the immune system in patients with HIV disease.[22]

Our study group maintained relatively stable laboratory values (including T-helper cell number, total white blood cell count, and hematocrit) during a thirty-month period while following this protocol. The mean T-suppressor number also rose by 27 percent. An increase in this value has been observationally linked to long-term survival in AIDS patients.[23]

It is our hope that intervening in a comprehensive fashion (as defined by this protocol) may enhance the immune system's ability to suppress viral activity. If this allows a greater length of time before the initiation of antiviral therapy, the high cost and potential for side effects inherent in the long-term administration of these drugs might be postponed. If nonpharmacologic measures initially prove unsuccessful as indicated by a declining trend in the T-helper cell number or clinical status, pharmacologic suppression could then be initiated.

In summary, our study sought to observe the ability of an early interventional program of nonpharmacologic therapies to support an HIV-positive individual's immune system. Although the data we have presented here are from a small pilot study containing too few patients from which to draw definitive conclusions, our experience with a standardized, nonpharmacologic, behaviorally oriented program indicates a potential beneficial effect on delaying the decline of functional status and T-helper cell counts in HIV-seropositive gay men. A larger, randomized, and controlled study of this approach is currently being designed to determine if this intervention may provide benefit when utilized as an adjunct to conventional therapies.

Jon D. Kaiser, M.D.
Department of Family Practice
California-Pacific Medical Center
San Francisco, California

This study received invaluable assistance from the efforts of three other researchers:

Elizabeth Donegan, M.D.
Associate Professor
Department of Laboratory Medicine
University of California Medical School
San Francisco, California

Dean Ornish, M.D.
Preventive Medicine Research Institute
Sausalito, California

Steven Sparler, Researcher
Preventive Medicine Research Institute
Sausalito, California

Table 1

PATIENT	AGE	BASELINE T-4	30-MONTH T-4	% CHANGE	AZT USE	SYMPTOMS AT 30 MONTHS
1	30	234	520	+122	no	none
2	50	362	273	−25	no	none
3	42	775	665	−14	no	none
4	42	187	187	0	no	none
5	38	138	36	−74	yes	weight loss
6	35	248	207	−17	no	none
7	39	863	1,000	+16	no	none
8	44	222	80	−64	yes	none
9	40	617	532	−14	no	none
10	59	432	408	−6	no	none
Mean Values:	42	407.8	390.8	−4.1		

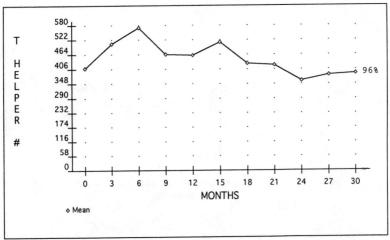

Figure 1

Figure 2

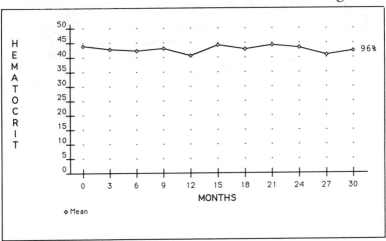

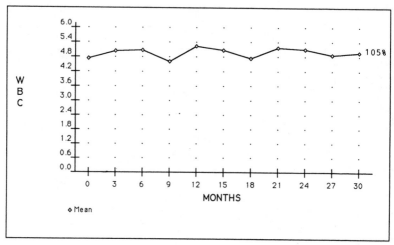

Figure 3

Figure 4

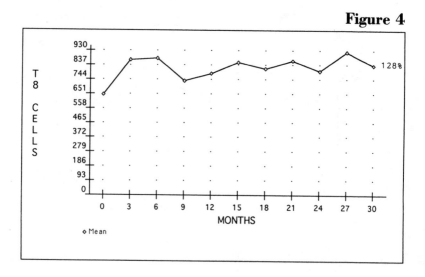

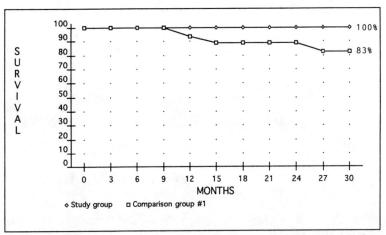

Figure 5

Figure 6

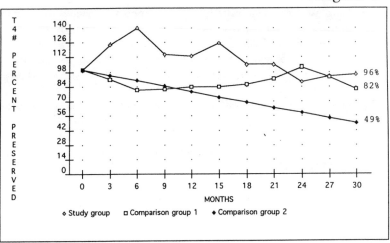

NOTES

FOR STUDY RESULTS

1. Scevola, D.; Barbarini, G.; Zambelli, A.; and Bottari, G. 1989. Nutritional status in AIDS patients (abstract). In *Proceedings of the Fifth International Conference on AIDS,* 465.
2. Moseson, M. 1986. Nutrition and AIDS. *Nutr. Res.* 6:729–30.
3. Grossman, C. 1985. Interactions between the gonadal steroids and the immune system. *Science* 227:257–67.
4. Riley, V. 1981. Psychoneuroendocrine influences on immunocompetence and neoplasia. *Science* 202:1100–9.
5. LaPerriere, A. R., et al. 1990. Exercise intervention attenuates emotional distress and natural killer cell decrements following notification of positive serologic status for HIV-1. *Biofeedback Self Regulation* 15:229–42.
6. Lang, W., et al. 1989. Patterns of T lymphocyte changes with human immunodeficiency virus infection: From seroconversion to the development of AIDS. *AIDS* 11:63–9.
7. Hickey, M. S. and K. E. Weaver. 1988. Nutritional management of patients with ARC or AIDS. *Gastroenterology Clinics of North America* 17(3):535–61.
8. Chlebowski, R. T. Significance of altered nutritional status in acquired immunodeficiency syndrome (AIDS). *Nutrition and Cancer* 7(1): 85–91.
9. Chandra, R. K. 1983. Nutrition, immunity and infection: Present knowledge and future directions. *Lancet* 1:688.
10. Position Paper No. 89-03, Position of the American Dietetic Association: Nutrition intervention in the treatment of human immunodeficiency virus infection. *Journal of the American Dietetic Association, ADA Reports.* 839–41.
11. Winick, M., et al. 1989. Task force on nutrition support in AIDS—

Guidelines for nutrition support in AIDS, *Nutrition* 5(1):39–46.
12. Colman, N., and Grossman, F. 1987. Nutritional factors in epidemic Kaposi's sarcoma. *Seminars in Oncology* 14:54.
13. Levy, J. A. 1982. *Nutrition and the Immune System: Basic and Clinical Immunology.* 4th ed. Los Altos, CA: Lange Medical Publications.
14. Nutrition and HIV infection. Summary paper prepared for the Food and Drug Administration by the life sciences research office of the Federation of American Societies for Experimental Biology, Nov 1990.
15. Prinz, W., et al. 1977. The effect of ascorbic acid on some parameters of the human immunological defense system. *Int. J. of Vitam. Nutr. Res.* 47(3):248–57.
16. Kennes, B., et al. 1983. Effect of vitamin C supplements on cell-mediated immunity in old people. *Gerontology* 29(5):305–310.
17. Harakeh, S.; Jariwalla, R.; and Pauling, L. 1990. Suppression of human immunodeficiency virus replication by ascorbate in chronically and acutely infected cells. *Proceeds of the National Academy of Sciences.* 87:7245–7249.
18. Dharmananda, S. 1987. Chinese herbal therapies for the treatment of immunodeficiency syndromes. *Oriental Healing Arts Intl. Bull.* 12:24–38.
19. Sun, Y.; Chang, Y. H.; and Yu, G. Q. 1981. Effect of Fu Zheng therapy in the management of malignant diseases. *Chinese Med. J.* 61:97–101.
20. Chu, D.T., et al. 1988. Fractionated extract of astragalus membranaceus, a Chinese medicinal herb, potentiates LAK cell cytotoxicity generated by a low dose of recombinant interleukin-2. *J. Clin. Lab. Immunol.* 26(4):183–7.
21. Chu, D. T.; Wong, W.; and Mavligit, G. 1988. Immunotherapy with Chinese herbs: Reversal of cyclophosphamide-induced immune suppression by administration of fractionated astragalus membranaceus in vivo. *J. Clin. Lab. Immunol.* 25:125–29.
22. LaPerriere, A. R., et al. 1990. Exercise intervention attenuates emotional distress and natural killer cell decrements following notification of positive serologic status for HIV-1. *Biofeedback Self Regulation* 15:229–42.
23. Vanham, G., et al. 1991. Subset markers of CD8(+) cells and their relation to enhanced cytotoxic T-cell activity during human immunodeficiency virus infection. *J. Clin. Immunol.* 11:345–56.

REFERENCES

Chapter 1

1. Centers for Disease Control. 1992. HIV/AIDS surveillance report.
2. Haseltine, W. A., et al. 1988. The molecular biology of the AIDS virus. *Scientific American* 259(4):52–62.

Chapter 3

1. Lemp, G. F., et al. 1990. Survival trends for patients with AIDS. *JAMA* 263:402–6.
2. National Research Council. 1974. *Recommended dietary allowances.* Washington, D.C.: National Academy of Sciences.
3. Sanchez, A., et al. 1973. Role of sugars in human neutrophilic phagocytosis. *Am. J. Clin. Nutr.* 26:180.
4. Bernstein, J., et al. 1977. Depression of lymphocyte transformation following oral glucose ingestion. *Am. J. Clin. Nutr.* 30:613.
5. Jacobsen, B. K., and Hansen, V. 1988. Caffeine and health (letter). *Brit. Med. J.* 296:291.
6. Riddick, H., U.S. Dept. of Agriculture. Personal conversation, May 1991.
7. U.S. Department of Agriculture, Nutrition Monitoring Division. 1986. National food consumption survey. Washington, D.C.: GPO.
8. Halsted, C. H., and Rucker, R. B. *Nutrition and the origins of disease.* Academic Press, 1989.
9. Werbach, M. *Nutritional Influences on Illness.* Tarzana, CA: Third Line Press, 1988.
10. Levy, J. A. 1982. *Nutrition and the immune system: Basic and clinical immunology.* 4th ed. Los Altos, CA: Lange Medical Publications.

11. Alexander, M., et al. 1985. Oral beta carotene can increase the OKT4+ cells in human blood. *Immunol. Lett.* 9:221–24.
12. Watson, R. R., ed. 1984. *Nutrition, disease resistance and immune function.* Marcel Dekker.
13. Cohen, B., et al. 1979. Reversal of postoperative immunosuppression in man by vitamin A. *Surg. Gynecol. Obstet.* 149:658–623.
14. Chandra, R. K. 1986. Nutrition and immunity—basic considerations. Part 1. *Contemp. Nutr.* 11.
15. Nuwayri-Salti, N., and Murad, T. 1985. Immunologic and anti-immunosuppressive effects of vitamin A. *Pharmacol.* 30:181–7.
16. Castleman, M. 1987. *Cold cures.* Fawcett.
17. Harakeh, S.; Jariwalla, R.; and Pauling, L. 1990. Suppression of human immunodeficiency virus replication by ascorbate in chronically and acutely infected cells. *Proc. Natl. Acad. Sci. USA.* 87:7245–9.
18. Meydani, S., et al. 1990. Vitamin E supplementation enhances cell-mediated immunity in healthy elderly subjects. *Am. J. Clin. Nutr.* 52:557–63.
19. Prasad, J. S. 1980. Effect of vitamin E supplementation on leukocyte function. *Am. J. Clin. Nutr.* 33:606–8.
20. Beisel, W. R., et al. 1981. Single nutrient effects on immunologic functions. *JAMA* 245:53–8.
21. Lim, T. S., et al. 1981. Effect of vitamin E on cell-mediated immune responses and serum corticosteroids in young and maturing mice. *Immunol.* 44:289.
22. The effect of vitamin E on immune responses. 1987. *Nutr. Rev.* 45:27–9.
23. Mowrey, D. B. 1986. *The scientific validation of herbal medicine.* Cormorant Books.
24. Tierra, M. 1983. *The way of herbs.* New York, NY: Washington Square Press.
25. Green, J. 1991. *The male herbal.* Freedom, CA: The Crossing Press.
26. Tragni, E., et al. 1985. Evidence from two classic irritation tests for an anti-inflammatory action of a natural extract, Echinacina B. *Food Chem. Toxicol.* 23:317–9.
27. Wacker, A., and Hilbig, A. 1978. Virus inhibition by Echinacea purpurea. *Planta Medica* 33:89–102.
28. Kulkarni, S. K., et al. 1972. Pharmacological investigations of berberine sulphate. *Jap. J. Pharmacol.* 22:11–6.
29. Dutta, N. K., and Panse, M. V. 1962. Usefulness of berberine in the treatment of cholera. *Ind. J. Med. Res.* 50:732–6.
30. Lahiri, S. C., and Dutta, N. K. 1967. Berberine and chloramphenicol

in the treatment of cholera and severe diarrhea. *J. Ind. Med. Assn.* 48:1–11.

31. Hunan Medical College. 1980. Garlic in crypotococcal meningitis: A preliminary report of 21 cases. *Chinese Med. J.* 93:123–6.

32. Dharmananda, S. 1987. Chinese herbal therapies for the treatment of immunodeficiency syndromes. *Oriental Healing Arts Intl. Bull.* 12:24–38.

33. Kou-sheng L., Chang P.W.H. 1950. In vitro antibacterial activity of some common Chinese herbs on gram negative intestinal pathogens. *Chinese Medical Journal* 68:307–312.

34. Young, M. Chinese herbal therapies and HIV infection: A clinical report. Reprints available from the Institute for Traditional Medicine, Portland, OR; (503) 233-4907.

35. Chu, D.; Wong, W.; and Mavligit, G. 1988. Immunotherapy with Chinese medicinal herbs. Immune restoration of local xenogenic graft-versus-host reaction in cancer patients by fractionated Astragalus membraneceus in vitro. *J. Clin. Lab. Immunol.* 25:119–23.

36. Chu, D.; Wong, W.; and Mavligit, G. 1988. Immunotherapy with Chinese medicinal herbs. Reversal of cyclophosphamide-induced immune suppression by administration of fractionated Astragalus membranaceus in vivo. *J. Clin. Lab. Immunol.* 25:125–9.

37. Chu, D.; Wong, W.; LaPushin, R.; and Mavligit, G. 1988. Fractionated extract of Astragalus membranaceus, a Chinese medicinal herb, potentiates LAK cell cytotoxicity generated by a low dose of recombinant interleukin-2. *J. Clin. Lab. Immunol.* 26:183–7.

38. Zhao, K. S., et al. 1990. Enhancement of the immune response in mice by Astragalus membranaceus extracts. *Immunopharmacol.* 20:225–34.

39. LaPerriere, A. R., et al. 1990. Exercise intervention attenuates emotional distress and natural killer cell decrements following notification of positive serologic status for HIV-1. *Biofeedback Self Regulation* 15:229–42.

40. Kusnecov, A. V., et al. 1992. Decreased herpes simplex viral immunity and enhanced pathogenesis following stressor administration in mice. *J. Neuroimmunol.* 38:129–37.

41. Glaser, R., et al. 1992. Stress-induced modulation of the immune response to recombinant hepatitis B vaccine. *Psychosom. Med.* 54:22–9.

42. Bonneau, R., et al. 1991. Stress-induced suppression of herpes simplex virus (HSV-specific cytotoxic T lymphocyte and natural killer cell activity and enhancement of acute pathogenesis following local HSV infection. *Brain, Behavior and Immunity* 5:170–92.

Chapter 4

1. Temoshok L. 1988. Psychoimmunology and AIDS. *Advances in Biochemical Psychopharmacology* 4:187–97.
2. Blaney, N. T.; Goodkin, K.; Morgan, R. O.; et al. A stress-moderator model of distress in early HIV-1 infection: Concurrent analysis of life events, hardiness and social support. *Journal of Psychosomatic Research* 35:297–305.
3. Riley, V. 1981. Psychoneuroendocrine influences on immunocompetence and neoplasia. *Science* 212:1100–09.
4. Achterberg, J., and Lawlis, G. F. 1978. *Imagery of disease.* Champaign, IL: Institute for Personality and Ability Testing.
5. Antoni, M. H., and Goodkin, K. 1988. Host moderator variables in the promotion of cervical neoplasia. *Journal of Psychosomatic Research* 32:327–38.
6. Seigel, B. 1986. *Love, medicine and miracles.* New York: Harper and Row.
7. Speigel, D.; Bloom, J. R.; Kraemer, H. C.; and Gottheil, E. 1989. Effect of psychosocial treatment on survival of patients with metastatic breast cancer. *Lancet* 2:888–91.

Chapter 5

1. Friedman, Y., et al. 1991. Long-term survival of patients with AIDS, Pneumocystis carinii pneumonia, and respiratory failure. *JAMA* 266:89–92.
2. Stites, D., et al. 1989. Lymphocyte subset analysis to predict progression to AIDS in a cohort of homosexual men in San Francisco. *Clin. Immunol. Immunopathol.* 52:96–103.
3. Volberding, P., et al. 1990. Zidovudine in asymptomatic human immunodeficiency virus infection: A controlled trial in persons with fewer than 500 CD4 + cells/mm³. *New Engl. J. Med.* 322:941–9.
4. Moss, A., et al. 1988. Seropositivity for HIV and the development of AIDS or AIDS-related condition: Three-year follow-up of the San Francisco General Hospital cohort. *Br. Med. J.* 296:745–50.
5. Fischl, M., et al. 1987. The efficacy of AZT in the treatment of patients with AIDS and AIDS-related complex: A double-blind, placebo-controlled trial. *New Engl. J. Med.* 317:185–91.
6. Pinching, A. et al. 1989. Clinical experience with zidovudine for

patients with acquired immunodeficiency syndrome and acquired immunodeficiency syndrome-related complex. *J. Infect.* 18:33–40.

7. Yarchoan, R., et al. 1988. Long-term administration of 3'-azido-2', 3'-dideoxythymidine to patients with AIDS-related neurological disease. *Ann. Neurol.* 23 (suppl.):S82–7.

8. Pottage, J., Jr., et al. 1989. Treatment of human immunodeficiency virus-related thrombocytopenia with zidovudine. *JAMA* 260:3045–8.

9. Richman, D., et al. 1987. The toxicity of azidothymidine (AZT) in the treatment of patients with AIDS and AIDS-related complex. *New Engl. J. Med.* 317:192–7.

10. Walker, R., et al. 1988. Anemia and erythropoiesis in patients with the acquired immunodeficiency syndrome (AIDS) and Kaposi sarcoma treated with zidovudine. *Ann. Int. Med.* 108:372–6.

11. Fischl, M., et al. 1990. Recombinant human erythropoietin for patients with AIDS treated with zidovudine. *New Engl. J. Med.* 322:1488–93.

12. Moore, R., et al. 1991. Non-Hodgkin's lymphoma in patients with advanced HIV infection treated with zidovudine. *JAMA* 265:2208–11.

13. Larder, B., et al. 1989. HIV with reduced sensitivity to zidovudine (AZT) isolated during prolonged therapy. *Science* 243:1731–4.

14. Fischl, M. 1991. New developments in dideoxynucleoside antiretroviral therapy for HIV infection. In *AIDS clinical review 1991,* ed. P. Volberding and M. Jacobson, 197–214. New York, NY: Marcel Dekker.

15. Yarchoan, R., et al. 1990. Long-term toxicity/activity profile of 2',3'-dideoxyinosine in AIDS or AIDS-related complex. *Lancet* 336:526–9.

16. Butler, K., et al. 1991. Dideoxyinosine in children with symptomatic human immunodeficiency virus infection. *New Engl. J. Med.* 324:137–44.

17. Kahn, J. D., et al. 1992. A controlled trial comparing continued zidovudine with didanosine in human immunodeficiency virus infection: The NIAID AIDS Clinical Trials Group. *New Engl. J. Med.* 327:581–7.

18. Yarchoan, R., et al. 1988. Phase I studies of 2'3'-dideoxycytidine in severe human immuno-deficiency virus infection as a single agent and alternating with zidovudine (AZT). *Lancet* 1(8577):76–81.

19. Merigan, T., et al. 1989. Circulating P-24 antigen levels and responses to dideoxycytidine in human immunodeficiency virus (HIV) infections: A phase I and II study. *Ann. Int. Med.* 110:198–94.

20. Meng, T., et al. 1992. Combination therapy with zidovudine and

dideoxycytidine in patients with advanced human immunodeficiency virus infection: A phase I/II study. *Ann. Int. Med.* 116:13–20.

21. Preliminary Results of ACTG 106. Presented at the April 20–21 meeting of the Antiviral Advisory Committee of the Federal Drug Administration. Reported in AIDS Treatment News Issue No. 150 May 1992.

22. Leoung, G., et al. 1990. Aerosolized pentamidine for prophylaxis against Pneumocystis carinii pneumonia. A San Francisco community prophylaxis trial. *New Engl. J. Med.* 323:769–75.

23. Raviglione, M. 1990. Extrapulmonary pneumocystosis: The first fifty cases. *Rev. Infect. Dis.* 12:1127–38.

24. Pierone, G., et al. Trimethoprim-sulfamethoxazole for secondary prophylaxis for Pneumocystis carinii pneumonia in AIDS (abstract). Paper presented at Vth International Conference on AIDS, Montreal, June 4–9, 1989. T.B.O. 6.

25. Stein, D., et al. 1990. Thrice-weekly dosing of trimethoprim-sulfamethoxazole for primary and secondary prophylaxis of Pneumocystis carinii pneumonia (abstract). In *Programs and abstracts of the 30th Interscience Conference on Antimicrobial Agents and Chemotherapy, Atlanta, October 21–24, 1990*, 854.

26. Rodgers, P., et al. The effects of PCP prophylactic agents on zidovudine-induced anemias (abstract). Paper presented at Vth International Conference on AIDS, Montreal, June 4–9, 1989. T.B.P. 324.

27. Metroka, C., et al. Successful chemoprophylaxis for Pneumocystis with dapsone or Bactrim (abstract). Paper presented at Vth International Conference on AIDS, Montreal, June 4–9, 1989. T.B.P. 4.

28. Nettleman, M., et al. 1990. Cost-effectiveness of alternative regimens for secondary prophylaxis of Pneumocystis carinii pneumonia (abstract). In *Programs and abstracts of the 30th Interscience Conference on Antimicrobial Agents and Chemotherapy, Atlanta, October 21–24, 1990*, 853.

29. Blum, R., et al. 1992. Comparative trial of dapsone versus trimethoprim/sulfamethoxazole for primary prophylaxis of *Pneumocystis carinii* pneumonia, Journal of AIDS, 5:341–347.

30. Israelski, D., et al. Prevalence of infection with Toxoplasma gondii in a cohort of homosexual men (abstract). 1990. In *Programs and abstracts of the 30th Interscience Conference on Antimicrobial Agents and Chemotherapy, Atlanta, October 21–24, 1990*, 115.

31. Nicholas, P., et al. Trimethoprim-sulfamethoxizole in the prevention of cerebral Toxoplasmosis (abstract). Paper presented at VIth Inter-

national Conference on AIDS, San Francisco, June 20–24, 1990: Th.B. 482.

32. Derouin, F., et al. 1990. Activity in vitro against Toxoplasma gondii of azithromycin and clarithromycin alone and with pyrimethamine. *J. Antimicrob. Chemother.* 25:708–11.

33. Young, L. 1988. AIDS commentary: Mycobacterium avium complex infection. *J. Infect. Dis.* 157:863–7.

34. Hawkins, C., et al. 1987. Mycobacterium avium complex infections in patients with the acquired immunodeficiency syndrome. *Ann. Int. Med.* 105:184–8.

35. Havlik, J., et al. Clinical risk factors for disseminated Mycobacterium avium complex infection in persons with HIV infection (abstract). Paper presented at VIth International Conference on AIDS, San Francisco, June 20–24, 1990. Th.B. 515.

36. Seigal, F., et al. Rifabutin may delay the onset of mycobacterium avium complex infection in patients with AIDS (abstract). Paper presented at VIth International Conference on AIDS, San Francisco, June 20–24, 1990. Th.B. 515.

37. Gonzalez, E., et al. 1989. In vitro activity of dapsone and two potentiators against Mycobacterium avium complex. *J. Antimicrob. Chemother.* 24:19–22.

38. Inderliad, C., et al. 1989. In vitro and in vivo activity of azithromycin against the Mycobacterium avium complex. *J. Inf. Dis.* 159:994–7.

39. Fernandez, P., et al. 1989. In vitro and in vivo activities of clarithromycin against Mycobacterium avium complex. *Antimicrob. Agents Chemother.* 33:1531–4.

40. Dautzenberg, B., et al. 1990. Clarithromycin trial group: Clarithromycin clears Mycobacterium avium-intracellulare from the blood of AIDS patients. A randomized trial (abstract). In *Programs and abstracts of the 30th Interscience Conference on Antimicrobial Agents and Chemotherapy, Atlanta, October 21–24, 1990*, 1264.

41. Bozzette, S., et al. 1990. Successful secondary prophylaxis of cryptococcal meningitis with fluconizole (abstract). In *Programs and abstracts of the 30th Interscience Conference on Antimicrobial Agents and Chemotherapy, Atlanta, October 21–24, 1990*, 1161.

42. Jacobson, M., et al. 1988. Serious cytomegalovirus disease in acquired immunodeficiency syndrome (AIDS). *Ann. Int. Med.* 108:585–94.

43. Mintz, L., et al. 1983. Cytomegalovirus infections in homosexual men: An epidemiologic study. *Ann. Int. Med.* 98:326–9.

44. Follansbee, S., et al. Phase I study of the safety and the pharmacokinetics of oral ganciclovir (abstract). Paper presented at VIth Inter-

national Conference on AIDS, San Francisco, June 20–24, 1990. F.D. 91. ﹐

45. Sande, M., and Volberding, P., eds. 1990. *The medical management of AIDS.* 2d ed. Philadelphia: Saunders.

46. Phair, J., et al. 1992. Acquired immune deficiency syndrome occurring within five years of infection with human immunodeficiency virus type-1: The multi-center AIDS cohort study (MACS). *AIDS.* 5:490–5.

47. Maddox, J. 1991. AIDS research turned upside down. *Nature* 353:297.

48. Dunkle, L., et al. 1992. Stavudine (d4T): A promising anti-retroviral agent (abstract). Abstracts of the VIIIth International Conference on AIDS, Abstract # WeB. 1011, Amsterdam.

49. Anderson, R., et al. 1992. Antiviral effects of stavudine (d4T) therapy (abstract). Abstracts of the VIIIth International Conference on AIDS, Abstract # WeB. 1010, Amsterdam.

50. Whelihan, W., et al. 1992. Effects of D4T on neuropsychological functioning (abstract). Abstracts of the VIIIth International Conference on AIDS, Abstract # PoB. 3033, Amsterdam.

51. Redfield, R., et al. 1992. HIV vaccine therapy: Phase I safety and immunogenicity using gp-160 (abstract). Abstracts of the VIIIth International Conference on AIDS, Abstract # TuB. 0563, Amsterdam.

52. Valentine, F., et al. 1992. A randomized controlled study of immunogenicity of rgp-160 vaccine in HIV-infected subjects (abstract). Abstracts of the VIIIth International Conference on AIDS, Abstract # TuB. 0561, Amsterdam.

53. Falloon, J., et al. 1991. A preliminary evaluation of 566C80 for the treatment of Pneumocystis pneumonia in patients with the acquired immunodeficiency syndrome. *New Engl. J. Med.* 325:1534–8.

54. Araujo, F., et al. 1991. Remarkable in vitro and in vivo activities of the hydroxynapthoquinone 566 against tachyzotes and tissue cysts of Toxoplasmsa gondii. *Antimicrob. Agents Chemother.* 35:293–99.

55. Bratt, G., et al. 1992. A study of gp-160 vaccine in healthy HIV carriers with and without zidovudine (abstract). Abstracts of the VIIIth International Conference on AIDS, Abstract # PoB. 3036, Amsterdam.

56. Sutor, G., et al. 1992. Anti-CD4 idiotype vaccination of HIV volunteers (abstract). Abstracts of the VIIIth International Conference on AIDS, Abstract # PoB. 3042, Amsterdam.

STRESS REDUCTION AND POSITIVE
AFFIRMATION TAPES

The stress reduction tapes distributed to Dr. Kaiser's patients and used by the research study group are available for purchase through the mail. The three tape package consists of the following six exercises:

Tape 1: Positive Affirmations/Opening Your Heart

Tape 2: Loving Yourself/Your Inner Advisor

Tape 3: Balancing Your Chakras/A Trip to the Grand Canyon

Send $24.95 (plus $2.50 shipping and handling) for all three tapes to:

> HealthFirst!
> P.O. Box 865
> Mill Valley, CA
> 94942-0865

(CA residents please add 8.5% sales tax to your order. Thank you.)

You can be placed on our mailing list to receive information on speaking engagements and important research updates concerning this program by sending your name and address to the address listed above.

INDEX

A-80987 protease inhibitor, 190
Abbott Laboratories, 190
Abrams, Dr. Donald, 176
Achterberg, Dr. Jeanne, 81
Acidophilus bacteria, 45–46, 174, 179
Acyclovir, 166
Adrenal hormones, immune system and, 81
Advanced glycosylation end products (AGE's), 29
Advertising tricks, sugar and, 30–31
Aerobic exercise, 71–74
Aerosol pentamadine (AP), 157, 161
Affirmations, 96–102
AIDS
  definition of, 1n, 15
  long-term survivors of, 77
  survival statistics for, 15–16, 122–124
  See also HIV (Human Immunodeficiency Virus), dormancy of
AIDS Care Symposium (1990), 3
AIDS Clinical Trials Group, 147, 150, 152, 164
AIDS Treatment News, 184
Alan, letters of, 105–107
Alan, viral dormancy of, 201–202
Alcohol, 21, 32, 168
Allicin, 54
ALT liver function test, 131

American Journal of Clinical Nutrition, 1973 sugar study in, 28–29
Amino Fuel, 24
Amoebas. See Intestinal parasites
Anaprox, 175
Anemia, 129
  AZT use and, 141
  PCP prophylaxis and, 160
Anger, white-cell count and, 80
Animal vs. vegetable protein, 24
Annals of Internal Medicine, ddC study in, 151–153
Antibiotic herbs, 51–55
  echinacea, 52
  garlic, 54–55
  goldenseal root, 52–53
  myrrh, 53–54
Antibiotics, diarrhea and, 175. See also specific medications
Antigenic activation, 176
Antimotility agents, 175, 177
Antioxidant compounds, 39, 41
Antiviral medications, 134–154
  AZT, 2, 5, 42, 43, 46, 50, 125–126, 135–145
  combination therapy, 152–154, 191
  D4T, 184–186
  ddC, 50, 149–152
  ddI, 50, 143–149
  protease and tat inhibitors, 189–191
  recommendations for, 133–137

Anxiety. *See* Stress
Apollinaire, Guillaume, 102
ARC (AIDS-related complex)
    AZT and white blood cell count,
        142
    Comprehensive Healing Program
        and, 7, 14
Ascorbic acid. *See* Vitamin C
AST liver function test, 131
Astra, 8, 68
Astragalus, 59–60, 68–69
Asymptomatic HIV-positive indi-
    viduals, AZT use by, 138–139
Atovaquone (Mepron), 188–189
Atractylodes, 62–63
Attitude, immune system and, 79–89
Autoimmune process of HIV, 183
Azithromycin, 162–164
AZT, 137–143
    asymptomatic use of, 138–139
    benefits of, 144
    ddC and, 150–154
    ddI and, 153–154
    herbal supplements and, 50
    information about, 137–138
    mutation of HIV to counter, 5
    recommendations for, 125–126,
        135–136
    resistance to, 143
    side effects, 140–143, 145
    studies of, 138
    therapy of, 139–140
    toxicity of, 2
    vitamins and, 42, 43
    zinc and, 46

Bactrim (trimethoprim-sulfamethox-
    azole, TMP-SMX), 157–159,
    161–162
Barley-cabbage casserole, recipe for,
    35
Barley and rice, recipe for, 34

Basic and Clinical Immunology, 1982
    vitamin A study in, 45
Basic chemistry panel, 130–131
Bear Valley Meal Pack bars, 24,
    173
Beliefs, affirmations of, 96–102
Berberine, 52
BETA, 140
Beta-2 microglobulin, 128, 133
Beta-carotene, 39, 44–45
Beverages, 20
Bilirubin liver function test, 131
Black, Susan, 68
Black walnut tincture, 178–180
Blaney, Nancy P., 80–81
Blastocystis hominis, 177
Blindness, CMV and, 166
Blood sugar test, 131
Blood transfusions, 129
Blood urea nitrogen test, 131
Bob, viral dormancy of, 197–198
Body, effect of mind on, 80–83,
    87–88
Body temperature, viral replication
    and, 72
Bone marrow
    anemia and, 129
    suppression of by TMP-SMX,
        158
Breads and cereals, 19, 25–27
Breakfast, 20, 23
Bristol-Meyers. *See* D4T (stavu-
    dine); ddI (didanosine)
British Medical Journal
    beta-2 microglobulin study in,
        128
    caffeine editorial in, 31
Bronchitis, 182
Brown rice, recipe for, 33
*Bulletin of Experimental Treatment
    for AIDS (BETA),* 184
BUN test, 131
BW256U87, 166

Caffeine, 21, 31–32
Calcium level test, 131
Campylobacter, 175
Cancer
  AZT and, 142–143
  fu zheng therapy and, 67–68
Candida albicans (thrush), 27–28,
  165, 168–169
Carl, viral dormancy of, 192–194
Carotenoids. *See* Beta-carotene
Case histories, 192–205
  Alan, letters of, 105–107
  Bob, viral dormancy of, 197–198
  Carl, viral dormancy of, 192–194
  Charles, viral dormancy of, 202–
    204
  Dennis, viral dormancy of, 195–
    196
  Ed, viral dormancy of, 204–205
  Forrest, letters of, 109–111
  Gary, letters of, 107–109
  Jack, letters of, 116–120
  Jake, viral dormancy of, 200–201
  Jim, emotional healing of, 84–85
  Jim, viral dormancy of, 198–199
  John, viral dormancy of, 194–195
  Joseph, letters of, 114–116
  Kyle, letters of, 111–113
  Larry, spiritual growth of, 86–87
  Robert, heart and mind of, 92–94
  viral dormany of, 201–202
Castleman, Michael, 41
Catnip, 56–57
CBC (complete blood count), 129–
  130, 141
Centers for Disease Control
  AIDS survival rate, 15, 122
  immunization recommendations,
    167
Cereals and breads, 19, 25–27
Chamomile, 55
Charles, viral dormancy of, 202–
  204

Chemotaxis, 52
Chest x-ray, 133
Chinese Medical Journal, garlic study
  in, 55
Chinese tonic herbs, 57–65, 68–70
  astragalus, 59–60
  codonopsis, 63–64
  fu zheng therapy, 67–68
  ganoderma, 61–62
  licorice, 64–65
  ligustrum, 61
  practitioners specializing in, 59
  RESIST formula, 58, 65–67
  schizandra, 60
  studies in HIV-positive patients,
    68–69
  white atractylodes, 62–63
Chloride level test, 131
Cholesterol test, 131
Chronic bronchitis, 182
Chronic indigestion, 182
Chronic sinusitis, 182
Clarithromycin, 162–165
Clofazimine, 163–164
CMV (cytomegalovirus), 166, 175
Coccidioidomycosis, 133
Codonopsis, 63–64
Cofactors, 181–184
  parasites as, 176, 182
Coffee. *See* Caffeine
Cohen, Misha, 68
Cold Cures (Castleman), 41
Collier, Dr. Ann, 153–154
Color of Light, The (Tilleraas), 102
Community Research Initiative, 164
Comprehensive Healing Program
  for HIV
  case histories of, 192–205
  history of, 7–9
  model of, 2–7, 9–10
  private practice data about, 11–
    16
  research study, 206–217

Contemporary Nutrition, vitamin A
   study in, 39
Controlled growth, 4
Cooley, Dr. T. P., 148
Cracked wheat cereal, recipe for,
   34–35
Cross-linking of protein molecules,
   29
Cryptococcal antigen, 132
Cryptococcal meningitis, 165
Cryptosporidium infection, 175,
   178–180, 188–189

D4T (stavudine), 184–186
Dairy products, 20–21, 168, 171–
   172
Dapsone, 159–162, 164–165
ddC (dideoxycytodine), 149–154
   combination therapy, 152–154
   herbal supplements and, 50
   information about, 159–150
   recommendations for, 137
   side effects of, 151–152
   studies of, 150–151
ddI (didanosine), 143–149
   AZT and, 153–154
   dosage information, 148–149
   herbal supplements and, 50
   information about, 143–144
   recommendations for, 136
   side effects of, 145–146
   studies of, 146–148
Decaffeinated coffee, 32
Deep breathing, 72
Deep relaxation, 74–76
   healing hour, 89–91
Demargination, 73
Dennis, viral dormancy of, 195–
   196
Depression, white-cell count and, 80
Dharmananda, Subhuti, 58, 68
DHPG, 166

Dialogue between you and HIV,
   103–120
Diarrhea, 173–176, 182
   weight loss and, 172
Diet, 18–36
   alcohol, 21, 32, 168
   breakfast, 23
   caffeine, 31–32
   cofactor possibilities of, 183
   dairy products, 20–21, 168, 171–
      172
   diarrhea and, 173–176
   energy levels of foods, 21–22
   fruit, 19, 27–28
   Immune Enhancement Diet, prin-
      ciples of, 19–20
   positive motivation, 33
   protein, 20, 23–25
   recipes, 33–36
   sugar, 21, 27–31, 168, 172
   vegetables, 19, 24
   weight loss and, 171–173
   whole grains, 25–27
Diflucan (fluconizole), 165, 169
Digestive herbs, 55–57
   chamomile, 55
   peppermint, spearmint, and cat-
      nip, 56–57
   slippery elm, 56
Digestive system
   acidophilus bacteria and, 45–46,
      174
   ddI and, 145–146
   diarrhea and, 173–176
   weight loss and, 171–173
Dormancy of HIV. *See* Viral
   dormancy
Drinks. *See* Alcohol; Beverages
Drugs, natural vs. synthetic, 47, 49.
   See also Experimental therapies;
   Standard Medical Therapies
Duesberg, Dr. Peter, 181
Dunkle, Dr. Lisa, 185

Eating. *See* Diet
Echinacea, 52
Ed, viral dormancy of, 204–205
Emotional healing, 79–120
  deep relaxation and, 76
  faith, 102
  growth, importance of, 79–87
  healing hour, 89–91
  heart vs. mind and, 92–94
  letters to the virus, 103–120
  major illness and, 77
  positive affirmations, 96–102
  positive attitude, maintaining,
    87–89
  stress as cofactor, 183
  support groups, 94–95
Enatmoeba coli, 177
Endolimax nana, 177
Endura Opti, 175
Energy, deep relaxation and, 75–76
Energy levels of foods, 21–22
Ensure Plus, 173
Entamoeba histolytica, 177
Enteric formulas, 175
Epogen (erythropoietin), 141
Epstein-Barr virus, hairy leuko-
    plakia and, 170
Erythropoietin, 141
Exceptional patients, 88
Exercise, 71–74
Experimental therapies, 184–191
  D4T, 184–186
  Mepron, 188–189
  protease and tat inhibitors, 189–191
  therapeutic vaccines, 186–187

Faith, 102
Falloon, Dr. Judith, 188
Fatigue, 170–171
Fevers, licorice and, 65
Fiber, value of, 27. *See also* Whole
    grains

Fifth International Conference on
    AIDS, 176
Flagyl, 177–178
Fletcher, Dr. Mary Anne, 75
Flu vaccine, 167
Fluconizole (Diflucan), 165, 169
Follow-up laboratory tests, 133
Food, energy levels of, 21–22. *See
    also* Diet
Forrest, letters of, 109–111
Free radicals, 38–39
Fruit, 19, 27–28
Fungus infections
  candida (thrush), 27–28, 165,
    168–169
  cryptococcal meningitis, 165
  histoplasmosis, 165
  prophylaxis for, 165
Fu zheng therapy, 67–68

G6PD (Glucose-6-phosphate-dehy-
    drogenase) deficiency, 160
Gainer's Fuel, 24, 173
Ganoderma, 61–62
Garcia, Wil, 99, 102
Garlic, 20, 54–55, 177
Gary, letters of, 107–109
Gastrointestinal tract
  acidophilus bacteria and, 45–46
  ddI and, 145–146
  diarrhea and, 173–176
  parasites in, 175–180, 182
  preventing disease of, 26
  weight loss and, 171–173
Gay bowel syndrome, 176
Genital herpes, 182
Gentian violet, tincture of, 170
GGT liver function test, 131
Ginger, 20
Ginseng, codonopsis as substitute
    for, 63
Goals, importance of, 88

Goldenseal root, 52–53
Gonorrhea, 182
Goodkin, Dr. Karl, 81–82
gp160 vaccine, 186–187
Grains, whole, 19, 25–27
Green, James, 51
Growth, 79–87
    attitudinal healing, benefits of,
        82–83
    emotional self, healing, 83–85
    spiritual growth, 85–87
    techniques for, 87–89

Hairy leukoplakia, 169–170
Halsted, Dr. Charles, 37
Hands, healing touch of, 89–91
Harakeh, Steve, 42
Harvard-Amsterdam AIDS confer-
    ence (1992), 185, 190
Haseltine, Dr. William A., 3–4
Hay, Louise L., 102
Healing hour, 89–91
"Healing Meditations" (Garcia and
    Melton), 102
Heart vs. mind, 92–94
Hepatitis
    ganoderma and, 62
    licorice and, 65
    schizandra and, 60
    test for, 131
    vaccine, 167, 187
Herbs, 46–70
    Chinese tonics, 57–65, 68–70
    digestives, 55–57
    fu zheng therapy, 67–68
    intestinal parasite treatment with,
        177
    nervines, 57
    practitioners specializing in, 59
    RESIST formula, 65–67
    western antibiotics, 51–55

Herpes, 182
Histoplasmosis, 133, 165
HIV (Human Immunodeficiency
    Virus), dormancy of, 1–10
    achieving, 3–4
    case histories, 192–205
    cofactors and, 182
    combining natural and standard
        therapies for, 4–6
    comprehensive healing program
        for, 7–10
    data about, 11–16
    definition of, 6–7
    incubation period, 122–123
    model for, 2–3
HIVID. See ddC (dideoxycytodine)
Hoffmann-LaRoche. See ddC
    (dideoxycytodine)
Hot tubs, 73
Humatin, 177–180
Hydrastine, 52

Immune Enhancement Diet, princi-
    ples of, 19–20. See also Diet
Immune Enhancement Project, 68
Immune system, complexity and re-
    siliency of, 5
Immunity soup, recipe for, 35–36
Immunizations, 166–167
Immunology Letters, beta-carotene
    study in, 39
Imodium, 175, 177
Indigestion, 182
Infections
    licorice and, 65
    opportunistic, 181
    prophylaxis and, 154–167
    white blood cell count and, 129–
        130
Influenza vaccine, 167
Insomnia, ganoderma and, 62

Institute for Traditional Medicine
and Preventive Health Care, 58
Interleukin-2, 69
Intestinal parasites, 175–180,
182
Intestinal tract. *See* Gastrointestinal
tract
Intuition, listening to, 92–94
Inulin, 52
Iodamoeba bütschlii, 177
Iodoquinol, 178
Isoniazid (INH), 133
Isospora, 175

Jack, letters of, 116–120
Jake, viral dormancy of, 200–
201
Jariwalla, Raxit, 42
Jim, emotional healing of, 84–
85
Jim, viral dormancy of, 198–199
John, viral dormancy of, 194–195
Johns Hopkins University, PCP
study at, 159
Joseph, letters of, 114–116
Journal of AIDS
Dapsone study in, 159
gay bowel syndrome article in,
176
Journal of the American Medical Asso-
ciation, "Survival Trends in
AIDS Patients," 15, 122
Journal of Clinical Laboratory Immu-
nology, astragalus study in, 69

KAL supplements, 40
nutrients of KAL Multi-Four tablets, 48–49
Kaposi's sarcoma, 176
Ketoconazole (Nizoral), 165, 169

Kidneys
acyclovir and, 166
function tests, 131
Kyle, letters of, 111–113

Lab tests, 124–134
basic chemistry panel, 130–131
beta-2 microglobulin, 128–129
CBC, 129–130
chest x-ray, 133
cryptococcal antigen, 132
follow-up, 133
P-24 antigen, 127–128
sedimentation rate, 130
TB, 132–133
T-cell panel, 124–127
toxoplasmosis titer, 131–132
Lactobacillus acidophilus. See Acido-
philus bacteria
Lancet, ddI study in, 146–147
Larry, spiritual growth of, 86–87
LDH liver function test, 131
Letters to the virus, 103–120
Licorice, 64–65
Lietman, Dr. Paul, 190
Ligustrum, 61
Lipisorb, 175
Liver function tests, 131
Lomotil, 175, 177
Long-term stressors, 76–77
Love, Medicine and Miracles (Siegel),
87–88
Lung infections, 133, 156–161,
188–189
Lymph nodes, exercise and, 72
Lymphoma, AZT and, 142–143

Maddox, John, 183
MAI (mycobacterium avium intracellulare), 162–165, 175

Male Herbal, The (Green), 51
Malnutrition, 37–38, 129
Medical Management of Aids, The
    (Sande and Volberding), 181
Medical therapies, standard, 121–191
    antivirals, 134–154
    cofactors, 181–184
    experimental therapies, 184–191
    lab tests, 124–134
    natural therapies and, 2–10
    prophylaxis, 154–167
    survival rates from, 15–16, 122–
        124
    treatment of symptoms and con-
        ditions, 167–181
Medication. *See* Drugs, natural vs.
    synthetic; Experimental thera-
    pies; Standard Medical Thera-
    pies
Medicinal plants. *See* Herbs
Meditation, 75
    healing hour, 89–91
Megace, 172
Melton, George, 102
Meningitis, 165
Mental attitude, 79–89
Mepron (atovaquone), 188–189
Metabolic needs, HIV infection
    and, 19
Meydani, Simin, 43
MicroGeneSys Company, therapeu-
    tic vaccine of, 186–187
Miles Pharmaceutical Company. *See*
    Mycelex troches
Mind
    effect on immune system, 80–83,
        87–88
    heart vs., 92–94
Mineral and vitamin supplements,
    22, 37–45
    nutrients of KAL Multi-Four tab-
        lets, 48–49
    potential side effects of, 50

RDAs of, 47
    schedule for, 39–40
Mint, 56–57
Mongtagnier, Dr. Luc, 181
Motivation, diet and, 33
Mowrey, Daniel B., 51
Mucilage, 56
Murray, Dr. Byron, 54
Mycelex troches, 169
Mycoplasma infections, 181
Myrrh, 53–54

National Cancer Institute, AZT
    study by, 142
Natural vs. synthetic drugs, 47, 49
Natural therapies, 17–78
    cofactors and, 183–184
    diet, 18–36
    exercise, 71–74
    herbs, 46–71
    standard therapies and, 2–10
    stress reduction, 74–78
    summary of recommendations
        for, 17–18
    vitamin and nutritional supple-
        ments, 37–46
Nature, autoimmune process of
    HIV article in, 183
Nef (negative regulatory factor)
    genes, 3–4
Nervines, 57
Nervous system, toxoplasmosis
    infection of, 160, 162, 188–
    189
Nervous system side effects
    ddC and, 151
    ddI and, 146–147
Neutropenia, AZT therapy and,
    141–142
New England Journal of Medicine
    aerosol pentamadine study in,
    157

ddI studies in, 147–148
Mepron study in, 188
Nizoral (ketoconazole), 165, 169
Norbeck, Dr. Daniel, 190
Nucleoside analog medications. *See*
AZT; ddC (dideoxycytodine);
ddI (didanosine); D4T (stavu-
dine)
Nutrition. *See* Diet
Nystatin, 169

Oat bran tablets, 174, 179
Oatmeal, recipe for, 34
Oils, 20
Onions, 20
Opportunistic infections, 181
prophylaxis and, 154–167
Oral hygiene, thrush and, 168–169
Organic produce, value of, 27
*Oriental Healing Arts International
Bulletin,* Chinese herbal ther-
apy study in, 58
Otto, Dr. Michael, 190

P-24 antigen test, 6, 137–128, 133
Pacific BioLogic, 58, 67
Pancreatitis, ddI and, 145–147
Parasites, intestinal, 175–180, 182
prophylaxis program for, 179
Pauling, Linus, 41–42
PCP (pneumocystis carinii pneu-
monia)
AZT and, 138
Mepron for, 188–189
prophylaxis for, 156–161
Peppermint, 56–57
Peridex, 168, 170
Peripheral neuropathy, ddC and,
151
Peyer's patches, stimulation of, 26
Pneumonia, bacterial, 167. *See also*

PCP (pneumocystis carinii
pneumonia)
Pneumovax vaccine, 167
Pollution, 38–39
Positive affirmations, 92–102
Positive reinterpretation and
growth, 80–81
Potassium level test, 131
Practitioners specializing in Chinese
herbs, 58–59
Private practice data, 11–16. *See also*
Case studies; Comprehensive
Healing Program for HIV, re-
search study
*Proceeds of the National Academy of
Science,* vitamin C study in, 42
Procrit (erythropoietin), 141
Prophylaxis, 154–167
CMV, 166
fungals, 165
immunizations, 166–167
MAI, 162–165
parasites, 179
PCP, 138, 156–161
recommendations for, 155–156
toxoplasmosis, 160, 162
Protease inhibitors, 189–191
Protein, 20, 23–24
sources of, 25
Protein molecules, cross-linking of,
29
Provitamin A. *See* Beta-carotene
Psychological distress
cofactor possibility of, 183
major illness and, 77
See also Emotional healing
Psyllium seed husks, 178–180
Pyrimethamine, 162

Quan Yin Center for Healing Arts,
fu zheng study by, 68
Questran, 175, 180

Raw foods, 21
Recipes, 33–36
  barley-cabbage casserole, 35
  barley and rice, 34
  brown rice, 33
  cracked wheat cereal, 34–35
  immunity soup, 35–36
  oatmeal, 34
Recommended Dietary Allowances
  (RDAs), 37–38
Red blood cell count, 129, 141
Redfield, Dr. Robert, 186
Reishi mushroom. See Ganoderma
Relaxation, 74–76
  healing hour, 89–91
RESIST formula, 58, 65–67
  contents of, 66
  dosage of, 66
  side effects of, 67
Rest, benefits of, 172, 174
Reticulocyte count, 129
Retin-A lotion, 170
Retrovirus, HIV as, 2, 4
Rev (regulator of viorion-protein
  expression) genes, 3–4
Rice, recipet for, 33
Riddick, Dr. Howard, 37
Rifabutin, 164
Riley, Vernon, 81
Robert, heart and mind of, 92–94
Rockefeller University, sugar study
  at, 29
Rutgers University, organic produce
  study at, 27

Salmonella, 175
San Francisco County Consortium,
  164
San Francisco General Hospital
  AIDS survival rate study, 123–124
  Chinese herbal study at, 69–70
Sande, Dr. Merle A., 181

Sandostatin, 175, 180
Saunas, 73
Schizandra, 60
Science, stress and immune system
  study in, 81
Scientific Validation of Herbal Medi-
  cine, The (Mowrey), 51
Sedimentation rate, 130
Seizures, ddI and, 146
Septra (trimethroprim-sulfamethox-
  azole, TMP-SMX), 157–159,
  161–162
Serum creatinine test, 131
Serum erythropoietin test, 129
Serum ferritin test, 129
Serum folic acid test, 129
Serum iron test, 129
Serum vitamin B_{12} test, 129
Seventh International AIDS Con-
  ference, 153, 162, 163, 186
Sex, unprotected, 182
SFGH AIDS Research Group, 70,
  123–124
Shigella, 175
Side effects, natural vs. synthetic
  drugs, 47, 49–50
Siegel, Dr. Bernie, 87–88
Sinusitis, 182
Slippery elm, 56
Smoking, PCP prophylaxis and, 157
Sodium level test, 131
Somatostatin, 180
Sordean, Jay, 68
Soup
  recipe for, 35–36
  value of, 24
Spearmint, 56–57
Speigal, Dr. David, 95
Spiritual growth, 85–87
Standard medical therapies, 121–191
  antivirals, 134–154
  cofactors, 181–184
  experimental therapies, 184–191

lab tests, 124–134
natural therapies and, 2–10
prophylaxis, 154–167
survival rates from, 15–16, 122–124
treatment of symptoms and conditions, 167–181
Stavudine (D4T), 184–186
Steam rooms, 73
Steroid hormones, immune system and, 81
Stress
cofactor possibility of, 183
definition of, 74
effect on immune system, 81
energy and, 23
long-term stressors, 76–77
reduction of, 74–78
See also Emotional healing
Subconscious, reprogramming the, 96–102. *See also* Emotional healing
Sugar, 21, 172
advertising tricks for, 30–31
immune system and, 28–30
pharmaceutical industry's use of, 169
thrush and, 27–28, 168
Supplements
acidophilus bacteria, 45–46
diarrhea and, 174–176
liquid food, 175
nutrients of KAL Multi-Four tablets, 48–49
nutritional, 173
potential side effects of, 50
protein, 24
schedule for, 39–40
vitamin and mineral, 22, 37–45
Support groups, 94–95
Survival rates, 15–16, 122–124, 138
Sweating, exercise and, 72–73
Synthetic vs. natural drugs, 47, 49
Syphilis, 181–182

Tat (transactivator) genes, 3–4
Tat inhibitors, 189–191
T-cells
antiviral recommendations and, 135–137
attitudinal healing and, 82–85
Comprehensive Healing Program effect on, 15–16
number of, 6–7
prophylaxis medication and, 156–157
stress and, 81
T-help vs. T-suppressor, 124–127
T-cell panel, 124–127, 133
Temoshok, Lydia, 80
Temperature, viral replication and, 72
Tests, 124–134
basic chemistry panel, 130–131
beta-2 microglobulin, 128–129
CBC, 129–130
chest x-ray, 133
cryptococcal antigen, 132
follow-up, 133
P-24 antigen, 127–128
sedimentation rate, 130
TB, 132–133
T-cell panel, 124–127
toxoplasmosis titer, 131–132
Therapeutic vaccines, 186–187
Thrush, 27–28, 165, 168–169
Thymus gland, adrenal hormones and, 81
TIBC (total iron binding capacity) test, 129
TIBO (tetrahydroimidazobenzodiazepine) antivirals, 190
Tierra, Michael, 51–52
Tilleraas, Perry, 102
Tonic herbs. *See* Chinese tonic herbs
Total parenteral nutrition (TPN) 173
Toxins, cleansing of, 26

Toxoplasmosis
    Mepron for, 188–189
    prophylaxis for, 160, 162
Toxoplasmosis titer, 131–132
Transferrin saturation test, 129
Treatment Issues (Gay Men's Health
    Crisis), 184
Trimethoprim-sulfamethoxazole
    (TMP-SMX), 157–159, 161–
    162
Tuberculosis (TB)
    MAI and, 163
    skin test, 132–133
Tulane University, vitamin E study
    at, 43
Twinlab supplements, 40

U.S. Department of Health, Educa-
    tion and Welfare, vitamin A
    study by, 44
U.S. Department of Veterans Af-
    fairs, HIV study by, 14–15
University of Miami Medical
    School, stress reduction study
    at, 74–75
University of Texas, astragalus
    study by, 68–69

Vaccines, 166–167
    therapeutic, 186–187
Valentine, Dr. Fred, 187
Vegetables, 19, 24
Vegetable vs. animal protein,
    24
Viral dormancy, 1–10
    achieving, 3–4
    case histories of, 192–205
    cofactors and, 182
    combining natural and standard
        therapies for, 4–6

comprehensive healing program
    for, 7–10
data about, 11–16
definition of, 6–7
model for, 2–3
Vitamin A, 39, 44–45
Vitamin C, 41–43
Vitamin E, 43–44
Vitamin and mineral supplements,
    22, 37–45
    nutrients of KAL Multi-Four tab-
        lets, 48–49
    potential side effects of, 50
    RDAs, 47
    schedule for, 39–40
Volberding, Dr. Paul, 140, 181

Way of Herbs, The (Tierra), 51–52
Weight loss, 171–173
Western antibiotic herbs, 51–55
    echinacea, 52
    garlic, 54–55
    goldenseal root, 52–53
    myrrh, 53–54
White atractylodes, 62–63
White blood cells. *See* CBC (com-
    plete blood count); T-cells
Whole grains, 19, 25–27
Writing, expressing your feelings
    with, 103–120

X-rays, 133

Yoga, 75
You Can Heal Your Life (Hay), 102

Zand's Insure Herbal formula, 67
Zinc, AZT and, 46